Traveling Without A Spare

A Survivor's Guide to Navigating the Post-Polio Journey

WENZEL A. LEFF, MD

Copyright © 2011 by Wenzel A. Leff, MD

WAL Publishing LLC
Pullman, WA 99163

ISBN: 978-0-578-08843-3

All rights reserved. No part of this publication may be reproduced, stored in a retrieval system or transmitted, in any form, or by any means, electronic, mechanical, recorded, photocopied, or otherwise, without the prior written permission of both the copyright owner and the above publisher of this book, except by a reviewer who may quote brief passages in a review.

The scanning, uploading, and distribution of this book via the Internet or via any other means without the permission of the publisher is illegal and punishable by law. Please purchase only authorized electronic editions and do not participate in or encourage electronic piracy of copyrightable materials. Your support of the author's rights is appreciated.

Printed in the United States of America

Contents

Acknowledgments 1

PART ONE 3

Chapter 1
My Story 5
    At the Hospital 6
    Homecoming 11
    Off to College 13
    Medical School and Beyond 16
    Polio Weighs In Again 19
    A Broken Leg 22
    Moments of Stupidity 24
    Retirement 25
    Back Surgery 27
    Back Surgery: The Sequel 28

Chapter 2
The Big Picture: The Four Stages of Polio 33
    My Four Stages of Polio 34
    Medical Illustrations of Polio's Four Stages 37
        The Acute Stage 38
        The Recovery and Stable Stages 41
        Post-Polio Syndrome 42

Chapter 3
Viruses and Polio: A Primer 45
    The "Good Old Days" of Polio 45
    The Polio Virus in the Twentieth Century 47
    What the Polio Virus Is and Is Not 49
    The Site of the Invasion: The Polio Virus Receptor 50
    Having Its Way with Us: How Polio Multiplies 51

The Blood-Brain Barrier: The Last Line of Defense........53
  A Bit about Vaccination................................56
  Postscript: Moving Ahead with Polio Research 57

CHAPTER 4
The Acute Stage: A Fight to the Finish 61
  The Pre-Clinical Phase: The Incubation Period 62
  The Clinical Phase: All-Out War........................63
  The Immune Response: Mounting a Defense.............64
  The Inflammatory Response 68
  Factors Affecting the Battle............................70

CHAPTER 5
The Recovery Stage:
Returning to Optimal Function.......................71
  Reviewing My Own Chart 72
  Three Phases of the Recovery Stage......................76
  The Cleanup Phase: Cleaning Up the Battlefield 77
    Rebalancing the Electrochemical Levels 78
    Removing the Dead Cells 80
  The Reinnervation Phase:
  Giving Orphaned Muscles a Second Chance 82
  Optimization: Maximizing Our Recovery................85
    Building Muscle Size and Strength 85
    Remodeling 86
    Accommodation 88

CHAPTER 6
The Stable Stage: Apparent Stasis 91
  Function and Reserves at the
  Point of Maximum Recovery 92
  Natural Attrition of the Aging Process 95

Chapter 7
Observing the Battle:
A Fictional Review 97

PART TWO 115

Chapter 8
Post Polio: An Introduction 117
Manifestations of Post Polio............................118
Post-Polio Syndrome 119

Chapter 9
Weakness 123
Peripheral vs. Central Muscular Fatigue 124
Muscle Fiber Types....................................124
Muscle Fuel..127
    Availability 127
    Toxicity...129
The Making of an Impulse 130
Treatment and Prevention 132

Chapter 10
Pain.. 137
The Polio Component 137
Pain Comes in Two Flavors 138
    Acute Pain 138
    Neuropathic Pain 140
Holding Still...141
Disuse...142
Compensation 143
More to the Story 144
Dealing with Post-Polio Pain 146

CHAPTER 11
Tiredness... 151
Depression as a Cause of Tiredness 152
The Strain of High Alert 153

CHAPTER 12
Difficulty Breathing and Swallowing 157
Bulbar Involvement in the Acute Polio Infection.........157
Post-Polio Difficulties in Breathing and Swallowing 160
Breathing 160
Swallowing..163
An Ounce of Prevention 164

CHAPTER 13
Falling.. 167
Risk Factors and Falling................................167
Post-Polio Limitations in Breaking a Fall 169
Preventing Falls 170

CHAPTER 14
Exercise 173
Disuse, Overuse, and Finding the
Right Balance in Your Exercise Program..................174
What an Exercise Program Should Do 176
Increase Strength and Endurance 176
Improve Fine Motor Coordination 176
Enhance Flexibility....................................177
Discourage Osteoporosis 177
Basic Concepts of My Exercise Program 178
Swimming: The First Inspiration......................179
Kegel Exercises: The Second Inspiration.................181
Giving the Concepts a Try 182
A Cautionary Note 185
In Conclusion..186

CHAPTER 15
Weight Control 189
Calories Count...190
Dr. Leff's Egg and Toast Diet............................193
How Much Are You Burning? 196
Tips for Success 197

CHAPTER 16
Self-Advocacy and Post-Polio Support......... 201
Take the Lead: Help Educate
and Focus Your Team..................................201
Proceed with Caution: Snake Oil and Anecdotes 202
Find Strength in Numbers:
Post-Polio Support Groups 205
Optimize Your Post-Polio Life: A Review 206

About the Author... 209

Index... 211

Acknowledgments

It wouldn't be too much of a stretch to say that I've been working on this book since I contracted poliomyelitis in 1949. But I have certainly not done it alone. I would like to thank some of the many people who have made the writing of *Traveling Without A Spare* a worthwhile experience.

First, many thanks to my early readers for their invaluable feedback: Canute Barnes, Howard Copp, Nancy Gregory, Peg Kehret, Ghery Pettit, Jack Rogers, John Thompson, Shirley Voyte, Stacey Walters, and longtime friend and author Jerry Travis, whose thoughtful and thorough review was immensely appreciated.

I owe a great thanks to the many polio survivors whom I have had the privilege of meeting. Their courage, stories, and encouragement have given me the required fuel to get this book to the finish line.

My daughters, Lori Leff Mueller and Lissa Leff Griffith, have worked alongside me, lending their keen editorial eyes and enthusiasm to the writing process. Their lifelong acquaintance with me and my disease made them the perfect pair to help steer this book into being.

I would like to thank all my family and friends for their patience and unflagging support. All of my children and their spouses have contributed in ways large and small to bringing this book to fruition, and to enriching my life. And to my ten grandchildren: thank you for being a constant reminder of the great bounty of life.

Finally I want to thank my wife, Julanne, who has been my navigator throughout my entire post-polio adventure, and 57 years worth of life's ups and downs. I cannot thank her enough for her love, dedication, grace and humor – and her help in keeping me focused on the road ahead.

PART ONE

Chapter 1

My Story

It was a hot – very hot – July 16th in 1949 when I became ill with what was soon to be diagnosed as polio, or "infantile paralysis." I was sixteen years old and had spent the day working in a hot, dusty attic, bringing the wonders of electricity to an old farm home outside my hometown of Mobridge, South Dakota. On weekends and during the summer, I worked as an electrician's assistant. The Rural Electrification Act had just been passed, and we were wiring electricity into farm homes that until this time had had their dark hours brightened by kerosene, gas lanterns, or sometimes just candles.

After work, I went home, cleaned up, and had supper (in South Dakota you have supper at night and dinner at noon – especially on Sunday). I was picked up by three of my friends, and we cruised Main Street for a while and then stopped for a Coke. That night, I was not my usual peppy self, and my discomforts, which I thought were just the aftereffects of working hard all day in a sweltering attic, kept getting worse. As the evening wore on, I felt hot, headachy, and tired. Finally, I asked my friends to take me home.

The next morning, my symptoms had progressed enough that my parents took me to see the doctor. Our family doctor's son and a friend of his had just graduated from medical school and joined our MD's practice. The younger men examined me and decided to do a spinal tap. In my spinal fluid, they found white blood cells consistent with infection, and gave my parents the news: I had polio. It was a logical diagnosis, as it was summer and there were outbreaks of polio all over the country. My symptoms were typical of acute polio, and finding cells in the spinal fluid was the clincher.

Within two hours, I was on my way to St. Luke's Hospital in Aberdeen, one hundred miles away. I would spend the next four and a half months in treatment there, not returning home to stay until the day before Thanksgiving.

At the Hospital

At St. Luke's, they placed me in a room in the basement of the hospital; it was a makeshift facility to take care of the polio epidemic. The beds were high and fix-framed, with flat springs and four-inch cotton mattresses. Our cubicles were separated by movable metal partitions with crisp, white cloth panels. The ceilings were low, the lighting was less than perfect, and the walls were institutional green, but, as you might expect, the Sisters kept the floors and fixtures immaculately cleaned and polished.

My twelve-year-old roommate was another of the fourteen people in the hospital from my hometown of four thousand. His older brother, Jim, had been admitted the night before and was in the next cubicle in one of the two or three iron lungs in our ward. Once I was settled into bed, the lights were dimmed, and I spent the next hour listening to the eerie, rhythmic groan of the iron lung motors and pumps; the footsteps of the nurse who followed the trail of a flashlight as she went from bed to bed, checking respirations and pulses; and an occasional call for help. It gave me time to think. It became apparent that there were people who were a lot sicker than I was. I didn't feel well, but I could remember days when I'd felt worse. I thought about some of the others who were calling out or crying and said a little prayer for them. In time, I fell into a light sleep.

The next morning, the nurses wheeled me into Jim's cubicle to greet him. There was a flurry of nursing activity around him. Jim tried to breathe, "Hi," as the iron lung exhaled for him. All I could see was his head sticking out of the massive chamber. His neck was paralyzed. He tried to move his eyes to find me, but his eye muscles were paralyzed as well. Because he could not blink to moisten his eyes, the nurses were applying saline and Vaseline to keep his corneas from drying out and cracking. I'm sure that any vision of me he had was just a blur. When they finished caring for his eyes and cleaning his airways, they wheeled my stretcher closer. I could see that, although he couldn't move a thing, he was very busy just hanging on – which he did for another forty-eight hours. Jim was not the last of the patients from Mobridge to die before the week was over.

Because of my headache and my hometown doctor's report that swallowing difficulties had kept me from eating, the hospital staff initially worried about my having polio of the *bulbar* type. In *bulbar polio*, the polio virus primarily attacks the nerves in the upper portions of the spinal cord (the brain stem), leading to difficulty with swallowing, breathing, speech, and eye and facial movements, such as my friend Jim had experienced. Though Jim's infection was generalized, it was the bulbar involvement – the destruction of his breathing centers and swallowing mechanism – that caused his death.

In contrast to bulbar polio, in *spinal polio* the polio virus primarily attacks the lower portion of the spinal cord, affecting motor function in the trunk and extremities. In my case, the weakness in my extremities began shortly after I was admitted to the hospital. Initially, it was in the left leg, but it soon spread to the right and then I was no longer able to walk. Fortunately, there was no obvious progression of bulbar symptoms, and the doctors diagnosed me with spinal polio.

At St. Luke's, polio patients were treated with the *Sister Kenny Treatment* – a set of protocols originally designed by Sister Elizabeth Kenny of Australia. Sister Kenny was a self-taught nurse whose interest in physical rehabilitation began when she herself was injured at age fourteen. Decades later, after having provided care to accident victims and soldiers in World War I, she created a set of therapeutic treatments for polio patients. Her motives and rationale were not without controversy and were questioned by some parts of the medical community, especially in her native Australia. Although these treatments did nothing to stifle the infectious process, nothing else had either. For many, hers was a "don't-just-stand-there-do-something!" approach.

I was placed in moist, woolen hot packs from my feet to the middle of my chest, initially on a daily basis. I still remember the elderly aid reaching into the hot kettle with a long wooden stick, much like the one my grandmother used for mashing potatoes, and pulling out the steaming hot woolen cloths to wrap around my legs and chest. The hot pack treatments continued throughout the summer months of July, August, and into September.

The Sister Kenny Treatment also included exercise and frequent stretching of the muscles to prevent contractures. Many of the exercises were done in large Hubbard tubs filled with warm water, where the water's buoyancy facilitated attempts to move my weakened extremities. The therapists also stimulated my muscles daily with *sinusoidal treatments* – electrical muscle stimulation that caused the muscles to contract. All of this was done to help the muscles maintain strength and range of motion (and were in direct contrast to other treatments in vogue at that time that promoted the splinting of involved areas and led to increased stiffening and weakness). Even though they did not "cure" anything, Sister Kenny Treatments had a very positive effect on the outcomes of those who received them. By preventing contractures and reducing irreparable disuse atrophy, the treatments helped keep our muscles, which had lost their nerve supply, viable enough to accept the reinnervation that, unbeknownst to us at the time, would mark the next phase of our polio journey.

I was given vitamins – some by injection, others in the form of a big capsule that I could not swallow, so I had to chew it while a nurse watched to make sure I got the whole thing down. I also received daily shots of penicillin and streptomycin. Though we have long known that polio is caused by a virus and that antibiotics are of no benefit in a viral infection, in those days, neither Sister Kenny nor the doctors knew much about what was going on, other than that polio was caused by a virus (whatever that was), the virus was killing nerves, and without nerves the muscles would not work.

The benefits the polio patients gained from Sister Kenny's treatments were the result of her instinct rather than any scientific knowledge that she could have had at that time. But I give her and the physicians of that day credit. They worked with what they knew, or thought they knew, and some of it was good – very, very good.

While in the hospital, the only time I was on my feet was when I was "stood" at the bedside for a few minutes each day or when, after eight or ten weeks, I was walked by two attendants as part of my strength and coordination recovery program. Otherwise, I was either in bed or in a wheelchair until they started me on crutches some time in my fourth month.

As soon as my condition stabilized and the doctors believed that I was no longer infectious, they moved me from the makeshift ward in the basement to a regular medical floor. Because they suspected that my hospital stay would be a long one, I was placed in the third-floor "long-stay area," which was, in reality, the geriatrics ward.

In the geriatrics ward, there were only two patients who did not have at least sixty years on me. It was a very boring place for a sixteen-year-old boy to be. In the evenings, I would often go down the hall in my wheelchair and visit with the elderly patients, trying to amuse them in an attempt to entertain myself. One evening, after I had finished visiting with one elderly lady, she rang for the nurse and asked, "Does polio affect the mind?" The nurses thought it was hilarious that this lady, who was herself suffering a degree of senile dementia, asked that question. I laughed along with the nurses, but to this day when I do something that is a little foolish or stupid, I ask myself that question: "Does polio affect the mind?"

Not infrequently, in articles and in discussions about polio – even in my own post-polio support group – there is talk about the abusive way the medical staff treated those of us with polio. At St. Luke's, that was not my experience. My care was good and loving and appropriate for the understanding of the day. Certainly, there was crying and screaming: we were sick, lonely, and frightened. We polio kids missed our moms and dads and siblings. Because we were quarantined, our parents couldn't come into our hospital rooms to visit us; they couldn't hold or hug us when we needed them. Sometimes they were able to wave through the windows, but many parents lived miles away and couldn't afford to travel. My dad saw me once during my four months in the hospital, and my mother never was able to come. There was much we as patients and children did not understand, and also some we didn't want to understand. It was a very difficult experience, but not for lack of care. I am very grateful to those at St. Luke's who put their own well-being at risk to care for me.

Homecoming

My family, my town, and my school actually kind of celebrated me when I got home. A few weeks after arriving home on Thanksgiving, I went to a dance and shuffled around. It was obvious that my jitterbugging days were over. My ladder-climbing days as an electrician's assistant were over as well, so I got a job at J.C. Penney's as a showcard artist, making price and product cards, doing the window decorating, and clerking on Saturdays. Although I never was much of a jock, it was obvious that any athletic aspirations I might have had would not be satisfied, so I concentrated on music and school politics. I couldn't march well enough to march with the band, but as student director, I could walk alongside the band, where if I were a bit out of step it didn't matter. (Hey, I was in uniform, and girls, it seems, have always been impressed by a fellow in uniform, whether he was leading the band, playing quarterback, or wearing Navy blues.)

I had ten weeks of schoolwork to make up when I returned home from the hospital. I would not be telling the truth if I said that I studied very hard to catch up – "by hook or by crook" more accurately describes how I did it. In the end, I did catch up and graduated with my class. Typing was the only class where my polio caused me academic problems. Because of the variance in strength, coordination, and responsiveness between my right and left hand, my right hand often pressed the key prematurely so, for example, "to" would often come out as "ot." I managed to get to the required thirty-six words per minute by the last day of the semester, and passed the class.

By late spring of 1950, my legs were working quite well. I couldn't climb, run, or jump, but I could walk slowly on the level without fatiguing. My high school girlfriend lived about as far as she could from my house and still be within city limits, which served as an incentive for me to walk. I can still walk with the assistance of braces and crutches, but I have not run, skipped, or jumped since July 16 of 1949.

My first summer after leaving the hospital, I helped my Uncle John on his farm. He thought he could strengthen me by having me shock oats. Shocking oats involves collecting the oats that the binder had bundled and dragging and stacking the bundles in a special arrangement called a *shock*, consisting of about ten bundles. This arrangement kept the heads up and off the ground so they would be dry when the harvest crew came to thresh them. Sometimes I would stumble and fall. I would then have to pile two or three bundles on top of each other to give me the leverage I needed to push myself back into the upright position.

I didn't give it any thought at the time, but have since wondered what I would have done had I stumbled or fallen upon a rattlesnake while working for Uncle John. I couldn't jump, run, or even quickly step out of its way. Yelling for help would have been a waste of energy because I was usually working a mile or more from help. Fortunately, I never had to find out. I'm not sure how much that job helped me to recover my lost strength, but Uncle John's idea of therapy was definitely an example of South Dakota work ethic, and probably no less scientific than any other recovery program available at that time.

Off to College

Although I had made the decision to go to college, I didn't have any money. A few weeks before I was to start at Yankton

College, the manager of the Penney's store in my hometown made a call to the manager of Penney's in Yankton and landed me a job doing signs, window decorating, and clerking – the same work I had been doing at the Mobridge store. The job assured me of an income for my first year of college. That income – plus a job as a biology lab assistant and the $200 savings I had in my pocket when I arrived at school – got me through the first year of college. My mother slipped me a few dollars whenever it was available as well.

I financed my second year of college by opening the first drive-in restaurant in Mobridge during my first summer home from school. I called it The Nibble Nook. It turned out to be a little too successful. Four new drive-in restaurants were up and running when I returned home the next summer. It was obvious that Mobridge did not need a fifth. I sold my restaurant equipment to one of the new operators and headed for Wichita, Kansas. I signed on to a harvest crew and worked my way back to South Dakota, finishing just in time to start school again.

It was in my second year of undergraduate school in Yankton that I met my wife-to-be, Julanne. She played clarinet in the orchestra, and I played trumpet. She thought my jokes were very funny, so we got married in August of 1954. Actually, there was more to it than that. She was beautiful and brilliant, and she did appreciate my humor. I found her easy to talk with, probably because I did most of the talking. It didn't seem to bother her that I was always broke.

Julanne's dorm at Yankton College was locked down at 9 PM, except on weekends when it might stay open until 10 or 11 PM. (The term *locked down*, which seemed appropriate for the management style of the girls' dormitory in 1954, is even more appropriate now that Yankton College has closed its doors and become a minimum-security federal prison.) The dining hall was closed Sunday evenings, so Julanne and I made it a point to have dinner out on Sundays. "Dinner out" consisted of heating a can of chicken noodle soup in a beaker over a Bunsen burner in the biology lab. I'm not sure that the college would have approved, but I was a lab assistant, I had a key to the place, we did not use any electricity – I considered it a legitimate perk of the job. We found that saltine crackers from the cafeteria with our chicken soup made a great meal. It was not until two days after our wedding that I discovered that it was the only meal Julanne knew how to cook. (I feel compelled to note here that, to this day, Julanne belittles her ability to cook. In reality, she quickly became a very good cook and an excellent hostess.)

Throughout my college years at Yankton, I was still recovering. Polio recovery is a fascinating process that can continue for months or years after the initial infection. It involves both the inward and outward changes that we make to accommodate the impacts of the disease. When all of these elements are at their peak, we have reached the *point of maximum recovery*.

I can't say exactly when I reached my point of maximum recovery. I remember my friend David in undergraduate school had a brown, sheepskin-lined denim jacket that he wore all four years of college. By the time we graduated, we noticed that the left sleeve of his jacket was worn and faded from my clutching it to keep from falling when we were on ice or snow or just walking fast – suggesting that I was still experiencing some weakness and instability and/or just being cautious through the fifth and sixth years following my infection. David suffered a stroke several years ago while teaching chemistry at Northern Illinois University and has since passed away; I think of him often and hope that he realized just how much I appreciated that sleeve and his friendship.

I can remember feeling fatigued sometimes when walking the ten blocks back to the dormitory from my Saturday job at Penney's. It was a gentle incline, but uphill all the way. If my legs became a bit fatigued, I found a fence or a hydrant to sit on or a post to lean against for a few minutes and then went on. This, too, suggests to me that I had not yet reached my point of maximum recovery while in college.

Medical School and Beyond

I'm often asked, "When did you decide to become a doctor?" The idea of being a physician floated around in my mind for a number of years, but I also considered theology, music, electrical engineering, and a number of other things before I finally ended up in medical school. At Yankton, two of my professors encouraged me to pursue medicine and from then on did not let me look in any other direction. I remain so grateful for their kindly intervention.

The University of South Dakota had a two-year medical school. I applied there and was accepted, and Julanne got a job as a secretary for the medical school's Bacteriology/

Virology Department. It was time for us to leave Yankton and move to Vermillion, South Dakota, where the medical school was located.

I heard about an apartment for rent near the medical school and understood that they were hard to come by. Julanne was unable to go check it out with me, so I made the trip to Vermillion by myself. The apartment was on the third floor, but the stairways had good handrails, so I thought my polio could handle a third-floor apartment quite well. The most exciting thing about it was that it was across the street from the main library – I could see the library entrance from the living room window. Because there was some urgency about signing up for an apartment, I made the $25 down payment and rushed home.

The next weekend I took Julanne to look at my find. By the time she finished surveying the apartment, she was in tears. She had discovered that, unbeknownst to me, we would have to share a bathroom (twenty feet down the hall) with three other apartments, two of them with children. She also noted that the apartment did not have running water in the kitchen, nor a sink or kitchen cabinets. (It did have a colorful porcelain dishpan sitting on a doily on top of the dresser, however). In the end, we decided not to live there. It was probably a good decision, but it still bothers me that Julanne did not take a single look out the window to see the library as part of her evaluation.

Ultimately, we found a basement apartment three blocks from school. Instead of looking down at a library from the third floor, we had to stand on a chair or the couch to see whether it had snowed the night before. It was a nice place, and our landlords were good people. Julanne and our landlady visited and played bridge in the evenings while I studied and our landlord slept. More than fifty years have passed, and we still communicate with them two or three times a year. (I should also say that we found that the medical school had a library of its own – so in my two years at USD, I never did have to go to the main library).

After finishing our first two years of medical school in Vermillion, my classmates and I went in all directions to find medical schools to complete our third and fourth years. I was accepted at Washington University in St. Louis. It was and still is a great medical school. I finished my internship and one year of residency at Washington University's Barnes Hospital and then finished my last two years of residency at Henry Ford Hospital in Detroit.

Medical school was extremely competitive, and my internship and residency years were rigorous. At one point, I even sent Julanne and our two daughters back for an extended stay with my in-laws because I was never home to see them. By this time, I had apparently stabilized from my acute polio, both mentally and physically, as I did not feel the need to slow down to accommodate it in any way. On the basis of these recollections, and a number of others, I would say my point of maximum recovery came about six years after my acute polio.

Once I had reached that point, and for the next forty years, my energy was almost limitless. I could get by very well on five or six hours of sleep a night. I dictated my medical charts from six to seven-thirty in the morning and then made rounds at one or two hospitals. I worked in the office from 9 AM to 6 PM or later, and on Saturday mornings. Every fifth weekend or so, I covered internal medicine for seven or eight internists at two hospitals, ten miles apart. (During the first twenty-seven years of my practice, we did not have emergency room physicians, so when we were on call, we covered all emergencies that came in, day or night, as well). I often had patients with especially worrisome problems call me at home with brief reports at 6 AM; that way I could schedule an appointment or lab tests or arrange for prescriptions before the rush of the workday began.

I was happy and energized by the intensity of my life as a physician. Though initial signs of post-polio deterioration were surfacing during the final decades of that time, because of the distraction of my career, most of my recollections of them have been in retrospect. I do not believe my busy lifestyle practicing medicine accelerated my post-polio deterioration; more likely, it had the opposite effect. I have no regrets.

Polio Weighs In Again

About 1980, the hyperextension in my left knee was becoming noticeable due to increasing weakness, the stress of being on my feet all day, and the middle-age weight I had gained. I started wearing a brace on my left leg. This marked the first overt and undeniable sign that my situation was no longer "stable." Eventually, this first brace was replaced by a better brace, and then both legs were braced. Over time, I was fit with several new sets of braces, each an improvement over the last, but still heavy and clunky. Attempts at reducing the weight of the braces by using aluminum rather than steel supports resulted in numerous emergencies, when the brace would break, leaving me stranded. I started carrying an extra brace in my car and made sure I never left home without it. As my dependency on my braces grew, so did my investment in their quality. Today I wear braces on both legs made of carbon fiber and titanium, which is stronger than aluminum and half the weight of steel.

My braces were designed to keep my knees from hyperextending, or curving backward excessively, a condition called *recurvatum*. Some recurvatum (about 14 degrees) was necessary to lock my braces when I was standing and walking. If I did not get the braces locked, the knees would buckle, and down I'd go.

I remember one embarrassing episode that occurred while talking to a patient. She was sitting on the edge of the examining table, and I was standing, nonchalantly leaning against the wall and the light switch. I was actually a bit too nonchalant, and my knee braces were not locked. Suddenly my knees buckled, and I slid slowly to the floor, my back against the wall, turning the light switch off as I slid. How do you handle a situation like that? My patient, who had watched me slowly slide down the wall, was now sitting in the dark. Fortunately, I always was pretty professional about my office behavior, so I kept right on lecturing while getting up, turning the light back on, and sheepishly apologizing on the way.

I remember another polio-related incident that happened

several years before I started wearing braces. I was doing a pelvic examination on a patient in the emergency room. I raised the electric exam table up as high as it would go so I could do the examination while standing because the exam stool they provided me was on rollers and too unsteady for me to get on and off. The patient was draped, and my hands were gloved. I extended my left gloved hand toward the nurse who was to apply some lubricant. She squeezed the tube of lubricating gel too hard, squirting more on the floor than on my glove. A moment later, while positioning myself, I stepped into the gel. My legs were too "polio weak" to allow me to jump and reposition myself. I tried to resist the slide, but my muscles were just not strong enough, and my leg slowly slid to the side. I found myself doing the splits. My patient saw me slowly disappear, with my sterile, gloved hand held high, as I slid to the floor behind her sheet-covered knees – like the setting sun.

Over the years, I was amazingly resistant to other diseases. I don't think I missed more than two or three days from work during my first thirty-five years of practice. Had I not studied medicine, I could easily have assumed that this resistance was because of the massive doses of penicillin and streptomycin that I took while hospitalized at St. Luke's. Having studied bacteriology, pharmacology, and physiology in medical school, however, I realized that those antibiotics could in no way have been a factor. I was therefore fascinated to read the reports from the Warm Springs conference on the late effects of poliomyelitis of 1984,[1] which indicated that many polio survivors shared with me a post-polio history that was relatively free of other infectious diseases. Such apparent resistance, however, did not seem to diminish the risk for noninfectious, age-associated problems such as cancer and lung and vascular diseases.

A Broken Leg

In September 2003, I fractured my femur and underwent surgery. The fracture was especially interesting to me as a physician and a post-polio patient. It was actually a combination of two different types of fractures, occurring within a split second of one another. I will elaborate because I think there are several lessons to be learned from my experience – not the least of which is to avoid fractures!

I was taking my wife's van to the dealership garage to get a professional opinion on what I thought might be a steering problem. I parked the van about seven feet from the entrance to the garage. As I was getting out, I realized I'd left my walking stick at home. I contemplated three options: (1) trying to make it without the cane; (2) going home to get the cane and then returning to the garage; or (3) aborting the whole

---

[1] The First Research Symposium on the Late Effects of Poliomyelitis, May 25–27, 1984, was hosted by the Roosevelt family and organized by Drs. Lauro S. Halstead and David O. Wiechers. It provided an opportunity for a number of polio researchers and physicians to evaluate the complaints of progressive weakness and pain reported by people who'd had their acute polio fifteen to forty years earlier. It was at this conference that the term *post-polio syndrome* was coined and the conditions required to justify its diagnosis first outlined.

mission. I felt quite good and decided on option 1.

I made it to the door without difficulty. Actually, I remember feeling rather smug about how well I had handled it to that point. I then opened the door and paused for just a moment, noting that it was only another seven or eight feet to the garage manager's desk. As I started my first step, I felt what seemed to be a one-half inch "give" somewhere in my left leg and then I fell harder and faster than I had ever fallen before, landing directly on my left knee. Nearly immediately, it was clear that I'd suffered a fracture, and not merely a bruise or a strain.

The x-ray findings were most interesting. They showed a spiral fracture of the mid-thigh and then two lineal fractures from the joint surface of the femur, pointing directly upward and perpendicular to the joint surface of the knee.

While I was lying on the cool, cement floor of the dealership garage, I surveyed the area where I had fallen and could see no grease or surface projections that could have caused me to slip or trip. I have to presume that a slight twist as I stepped through the door caused the spiral fracture in the femur, creating the sensation of the one-half inch give as I took that step. When I fell, I landed directly on my knee, resulting in the two fractures extending up from the joint surface.

A spiral fracture is almost always associated with bone thinning (*osteoporosis*) rather than trauma, and it was in my case as well. Osteoporosis is relatively uncommon in men, occurring with a ratio of about 8:1 women to men. But my history of braces and more limited weight-bearing may explain my osteoporosis. Bone needs to be stressed and stimulated to grow and remain strong. Although I have led a busy life, once I entered medical school I never engaged in regular, weight-bearing physical exercise beyond that required to get from one place to another. Later, my use of braces, necessary to control the recurvatum in my legs and to allow me to stand and walk, also reduced the stress on the bones of my legs. All of this may have contributed to bone thinning and ultimately made my femur more susceptible to fracture.

My experience is one illustration of how post-polio patients may be more susceptible than others to some diseases or stresses that would appear unrelated to polio. In this case, the spiral fracture was associated with the osteoporosis that had resulted from disuse of my bones, caused in part by the braces that I needed to walk.

The other lesson from my experience is that, as post-polio patients, we need to use good judgment. We have to take into consideration our relative lack of strength, decreased balance and coordination, easy fatigability, and the like, when we make decisions. In my case, I made a bad decision.

Moments of Stupidity

When I was practicing medicine, I would tell my cardiac patients to avoid "moments of stupidity." For example, don't get out and help push your friend's truck out of a snow bank. A cardiac patient should know that that is more of a risk than he should take, even though he might be tempted to lend a hand to a friend in need.

I had a patient, Dr. K, with heart disease, who taught at the School of Veterinary Medicine at the university in our hometown. He was, I think, a bit offended that I should lecture him about moments of stupidity. After all, he had a doctorate in veterinary medicine and a number of other degrees. He not only practiced medicine, he taught the course. One day, I got a call as I was about to break for lunch: Dr. K was on his way over to my office and thought he was having a heart attack. When he arrived, he was quick to confess what had happened. He said that he was demonstrating to a student how to hold a calf while giving a shot. Apparently there is a very special way to hold the animal so it will not escape while being injected or examined. This time, however, the calf did break away. "Impulsively, I took off on a run to catch the critter," Dr. K told me. "After about thirty feet, I could feel my chest cave in on me with severe pain and shortness of breath. And all I could think was … this is a moment of stupidity."

A moment of stupidity is what led to my fracture. It wasn't as reflexive or impulsive as Dr. K's, but it was a matter of poor judgment – the effects of which I have had to pay for, and will probably continue paying for, for the rest of my life.

Retirement

Shortly before I broke my leg, I had retired from my medical practice. In search of ways to spend my new retirement time, I purchased a six-wheel drive Polaris All-Terrain Vehicle, thinking that it could get me into the wild where I could take a few pictures, pick a few berries, find a shore to fish from, and so on. A six-wheeled ATV should do that, but I found that ATVs were designed for a physically tougher sort than me, and modifications were necessary.

My legs were too weak to manage the ATV's brakes in the hilly, mountainous backcountry, so I installed a vacuum booster to reduce the amount of pressure I needed to apply to work them. I also rebuilt the brake pedal so my foot wouldn't slip from it when rough terrain bounced me around. I equipped it with a good rope, pulley, and fire extinguisher for emergencies. Mine was a two-seater, much like a golf cart, so I could have someone with me when I went out exploring the country. It was a great piece of equipment, and, with the modifications, I could manage it pretty well. It could go anywhere – and, unfortunately, it did.

The second morning of spring, before my ATV had had its first birthday, I arrived at the cabin only to find the yard gate broken, my shop door lock broken, and my ATV and its trailer gone. Someone had stolen my six-wheeled ticket to adventure. Though I was sad for the loss (and a bit disappointed in humanity), when the insurance money came, rather than replacing my ATV, I bought a small tractor with mower, rototiller, posthole digger, and front-end bucket.

Getting the tractor was a good idea. With the tractor I could be productive and still be doing something I really enjoyed. With the ATV, if I got stuck or fell, I could not get up or out without help, so with my post-polio weakness I always needed someone to be with me, and it is no fun to always be dependent on someone else. Though my new tractor was also perfectly capable of tipping me over, throwing me off, or getting stuck, my ten-acre playground of workable land was very visible from our house, so it would be easy for me to call or even wave in case of emergency.

Unfortunately, the land I had to work was very rough and rocky, and after a springtime of tractor riding, I began to experience back pain. At first, I was hopeful that it was exercise-induced and signified I was getting stronger and more fit. But by the end of the summer, the pain could not be ignored and had begun to radiate into my leg.

Back Surgery

My doctors ordered an MRI, which showed a *herniating disc* in very close proximity to my spinal cord. By the time the MRI was performed, the herniation was already interfering with the free flow of spinal fluid and threatening the cord itself. Even relatively light pressure directly on the spinal cord can cause paralysis of the organs below that nerve level due to interference with the cord's blood supply. What I was experiencing could result in loss of muscle and sensory function in the low back and legs as well as loss of bowel and bladder control. It called for prompt repair.

In early 2007, I was referred to a University of Washington orthoneurosurgeon for surgery. My local orthopedist and longtime friend did not want to touch me – too risky – he wanted someone with expertise in that location and that type of problem to do the operation. The surgery went well, and the disc pain was gone by the time I returned to my room; however, about five days following the surgery, a different back pain developed.

This new pain was a puzzler. It was obviously not related to the herniated disc in that it was diffuse rather than localized and did not radiate into my legs as the disc pain had. For the week or two before surgery and the few weeks after surgery, I was unable to exercise the already-weakened muscles needed to support and stabilize my back and legs. This disuse was the culprit, I am sure, and as a result, recovery from the disc herniation surgery was slow and less than perfect. With exercise and time, however, adequate recovery did occur, but I never did get back to a point where I could safely walk without crutches.

Back Surgery: The Sequel

About a year later, pain started again. This was very disappointing because, until my leg fracture, my post-polio time had been almost free of pain. Now it seemed I was never in the clear. This time the pain was in the left leg and across the back. I returned to the University of Washington, where studies showed that my *scoliosis* – the curvature in my lower spine due to the partial collapse of the vertebrae and discs in my back – had progressed markedly. After deliberation, we decided to go ahead with surgery to stabilize my back by fusing four discs together (L3–S1).

It was not an easy procedure. During the entire eight-hour surgery, I was face down on my abdomen. I was given six units of blood while I was on the table and another two the following morning. Post-operatively, they had difficulty stabilizing my blood pressure and I spent an extra twenty-four hours in intensive care before being transferred to the surgical recovery unit where I spent the next seven days.

At the end of that time, I was certainly in no condition to manage at home, but I was told that the rehabilitation unit was full and there would be no room for me there for at least four to six weeks. On the day of my scheduled discharge from the surgical recovery unit, however, God smiled upon me, and a team from rehabilitation arrived and transferred me to their digs where I spent the next three weeks.

The University of Washington Medical Center Rehabilitation Department was first class. The treatment was intense and appropriate, the people caring for me were knowledgeable and marvelous, and I hated almost every minute of my experience there. It hurt to move, and they made me move. I felt too weak to walk, and they made me walk. To make matters worse, my bowel took issue with the pain medications, necessitating that bold measures be taken to right the situation. These "bold measures" were not unlike a peacetime version of waterboarding – and I must say they were able to get everything they wanted out of me where all previous methods had failed.

The rehabilitation experts who treated me were just as eager to learn from my experience as they were to instruct and educate me. Those of us who have suffered from polio have spent years developing tricks and work-arounds to accommodate the residual defects left by the disease. It was refreshing and encouraging to be involved with caregivers who were not only genuinely interested in learning as much as they could about the unique mechanics of the post-polio body, but who also had such an appreciation for the resourcefulness we used in accommodating it.

My rehab was not all just healing the tissues that had been injured and my body accepting the metal placed in my back to stabilize it. I was a different person when I came back from surgery: I was foggy, lacking in memory, unable to do sequences of numbers, and unaware of date and time. My family and I laughed and made light of the confusing things I said, but I was aware enough to be worried about these mental problems being a permanent thing. I knew how to live (and even excel) with limited leg function and generalized weakness, but I did not want to live without the full use of my brain.

The medical team at the hospital reassured me that it was typical for anesthesia and pain medication to cause some post-surgical confusion, lack of memory, and difficulty organizing and calculating. (As a doctor I knew this already, but as a patient I wanted to hear it again.) I also had weakness more severe and more generalized than I'd had before surgery. I could accept that these symptoms were residual effects from anesthesia and muscle relaxants for a day or two, maybe three, after surgery, but I became doubtful when it lasted longer than that. I had planned to use my post-surgery recovery time to finish this book, but my head was so dull and my ability to concentrate so poor that I couldn't have written a letter to Santa Claus, much less a book.

I became depressed and diffusely weakened and lost motivation to get back into my exercise and get-well program. It was not until six months after surgery that I was able to conjure up a creative thought and another three weeks after that before I felt like I was getting back toward normal.

Since then, I have given much thought and done much research in search of a more plausible cause for my prolonged recovery. A number of factors had the potential to have played a part, and I have considered many possibilities. I do not know for sure, but what I do know is that I took a real hit.

My last few years have been a symptomatic hodgepodge: symptoms related to aging, joint pain, situational depression, trauma, surgeries … and possibly polio. Though the recent years in particular have not been easy, the medical scientist in me is happy to have had them in that they have allowed me to experience my life in Post Polio more completely.

This chapter has been my personal polio history. I wanted to start with it because it provides some helpful illustrations as you, the reader, learn more about polio, post-polio syndrome, and the post-polio period. I also wanted you to know that I am an author who has "been there and done that." I have survived polio, and, for those of you who are polio survivors, I am experiencing many of the same things you have been through or are currently experiencing with your polio, or that you may have to deal with in the future.

Does it make a difference to you that I had polio? I hope so. I remember that when I was practicing medicine I had a number of patients suffering with alcoholism who were reluctant to work with a counselor who was not a recovering alcoholic. I am sure it was not "a union thing"; they just didn't feel a counselor who had not lived through alcohol addiction could really understand what they were going through. Some of my patients with depression also found it hard to believe that a therapist could really understand how terrible they felt without having been through severe depression himself. You will see that, as a result of having lived with polio and its various manifestations since 1949 and having studied and practiced medicine since 1955, my observations, presentations, and interpretations will reflect both my internal medicine background and my life with polio.

CHAPTER 2

THE BIG PICTURE: THE FOUR STAGES OF POLIO

For most of my adult life, I lived in a state of denial; I was too busy and functioning too well to think much about my polio. I assumed that the worst was over – the polio infection was done – and that if any further insults to my health were to occur, as a physician, I could avoid, prevent, or control them. I guess I thought that I wouldn't let those "post-polio things" happen to me. But they came to pass, and here I am. Post Polio reared its ugly head and let me know the polio story was not yet complete.

In the following chapters, we will look at polio and its various manifestations more completely – more scientifically, if you will. With a better understanding of what happens to the body when first infected by polio and what then happens to it afterward, we might be able to temper or accommodate some of those post-polio things, enabling a life with less fear and more comfort and productivity.

The polio experience may be divided clinically into four stages: the *Acute Stage*, the *Recovery Stage*, the *Stable Stage*, and *Post Polio*. We will begin by looking at all of these stages as they are illustrated by my history and then dig a little deeper to get a more scientific understanding of each stage.

My Four Stages of Polio

My first stage, the Acute (infectious) Stage, lasted about three weeks, including an incubation period of one or two weeks that preceded the onset of any noticeable symptoms. It was played out clinically in that hot, dusty attic when I began to feel a bit sick. It continued while I cruised Main Street with my friends and asked them to take me home early. It persisted the next day while I was in the doctor's office where they made the diagnosis of polio, and while I was transported one hundred miles in the backseat of a Hudson Terraplane to Aberdeen for treatment. The Acute Stage also continued through the beginning of my time as a patient in the polio ward in the basement of St. Luke's Hospital.

The second stage, the Recovery Stage, started with the hot packs, stretching, and exercises at St. Luke's and continued for another five or six years, during which time the activities of my daily living and work replaced the more formal rehabilitation-therapy program of my months in the hospital. Despite the tremendous importance of the exercise and therapy programs, I will soon explain how most of the improvement of the Recovery Stage resulted from the *reinnervation* that was occurring behind the scenes – nerve branches sprouting from the surviving nerves, attaching themselves to some of the orphaned muscle fibers that were in the neighborhood, and reestablishing a degree of muscle function.

The exact beginning and end of my third stage, the Stable Stage, are not easy to pinpoint, but this stage was the period of relative stability that began about the time I started medical school and continued for over thirty years. I was busy, physically active, and productive. My recovery had maximized. I was able to work and play and compete. The limitations polio had left me with were acceptable. At this point, I thought polio and I had a deal, that we'd negotiated a settlement. Never, never did I think that polio might have more tricks to play.

But then came the fourth stage, tethering me once again with an onset of weakness, easy fatigability, and pain. The nerve sprouts that had given me back my lost mobility in 1949 were now failing, and that failure marked the beginning of the fourth stage: Post Polio. For me, it meant wearing leg braces, avoiding stairs, using handicapped parking, and investigating, and ultimately embracing, mobility options such as crutches, scooters, and more.

From my story, you can clearly see the four stages through which most survivors of paralytic polio seem to progress: the active, infectious Acute Stage; the slow rebuilding period of the Recovery Stage; the deceptively static phase of the Stable Stage; and the frustrating realizations of Post Polio.

Although the fourth stage, Post Polio, includes "post-polio syndrome" and seems to present itself as a new set of noticeable symptoms, in reality Post Polio may be the culmination of the first three stages in combination with the natural effects of aging. The nervous systems of polio survivors were severely compromised during the acute infection of the first stage of polio. The recovery process of the second stage featured miraculous – but somewhat less than perfect – nerve regeneration (*reinnervation*), which gave us improved functional capacity but still left us with depleted neuromuscular reserves. The impression of stability in the third stage was misleading, as it was in truth a very dynamic time of ongoing changes – including subtle nerve degeneration, further depleting our reserves. So when our polio history is combined with the neuromuscular loss that naturally accompanies the aging process, we end up with functional neuromuscular capacity that falls below critical mass – we cross the line from *enough* to *not enough*. Post Polio is evidence of this failure becoming overt, manifested clinically by the progression of weakness, fatigue, pain, breathing difficulties, and other symptoms.

Medical Illustrations of Polio's Four Stages

Now that we've reviewed the four stages of my polio, let's take a more scientific look at the nerve changes that were occurring at each of those stages.

In 1999, the Post-Polio Task Force published a series of illustrations depicting the effect of the polio virus on the typical motor nerve cell and its attachment to muscle.[2] The illustrations told the story of what happened and is happening to the nerves as a result of polio infection more clearly and simply than almost anything else I've seen or read.[3] A

---

[2] Post-Polio Task Force (Neil R. Cashman, Chair), Slides 10 through 13, "Peripheral Disintegration Model of PPS," *Post-Polio Syndrome Slide Kit*, (New York: BioScience Communications, 1999). The Post-Polio Task Force was a group of eight experts from the post-polio healthcare and patient communities whose mission was to raise awareness of and disseminate information on post-polio syndrome. The illustrations were part of a slide kit developed to aid in lectures to advance that mission.

[3] The slides illustrate the peripheral disintegration model of post polio, first set out by David O. Wiechers and Susan L. Hubbell in "Late changes in the motor unit after acute poliomyelitis," *Muscle & Nerve* 4, no. 6 (1981): 524–528. The theory suggests that these late effects of polio are related to the degeneration over time of the axon sprouts that developed years before, after the acute infection, to reinnervate muscle whose original innervations had been destroyed by the virus.

careful review of the images I've included here will give you a good basic understanding of polio infection and Post Polio.[4]

The Acute Stage

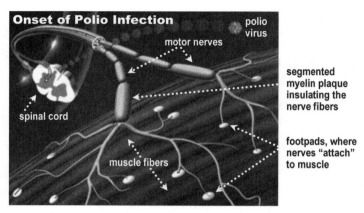

Figure 1: Healthy nerves and muscles as polio infection sets in.

The first illustration shows nerve and muscle at the onset of the polio infection; it is essentially a *before* picture. Figure 1 shows a cross-section of the spinal cord with two motor nerves emerging from it that extend to the muscle. Muscle movement is achieved through the process of *innervation*, whereby impulses are sent from the brain and transmitted through motor nerves to the muscles. You'll notice that the nerve fibers are covered with segmented plaques of fatty material (*myelin*),

---

[4] The original illustrations have since been updated and are now available at the website for Post-Polio Health International (http://www.post-polio.org/edu/hpros/task/CD/index.html). The images included in Figures 1-6 are based on these illustrations, with permission from Post-Polio Health International.

which serve to protect and insulate the nerve fibers. A healthy coating of myelin allows nerve impulses to be transmitted more quickly and discretely. You see branching of the motor nerve fibers into multiple nerve branches, or *axons*. At the end of each nerve branch is a *footpad* that is attached to the muscle fibers and through which the impulse is transmitted.[5]

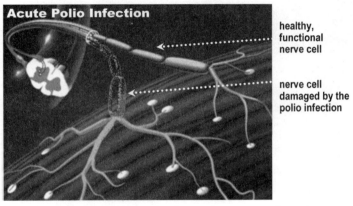

Figure 2: Nerves and muscle during the acute polio infection.

In Figure 2 the polio infection is in full swing. The primary thing to notice here is the obvious disintegration of the infected lower nerve; the nerve appears moth-eaten – if the nerve fails, its branches will fail, too.

---

[5] The footpad and the muscle fiber are not actually physically attached. Vesicles manufactured in the nerve nucleus are filled with a chemical called *acetylcholine*. Acetylcholine drips from the footpad onto the receptor site on the muscle fiber to give the muscle its direction.

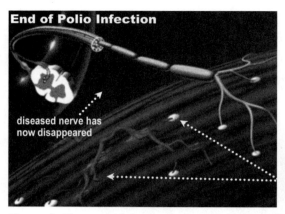

Figure 3: The end of the Acute Stage of polio infection.

Figure 3 is the *after* picture, depicting the full extent of the damage. Note that the infected lower nerve has now disappeared, having disintegrated completely. As we anticipated, the lower nerve's branches are gone, and the footpads, where the nerves attach to the muscle, have disintegrated as well. The muscle the infected nerve supplied is now paralyzed, as it is an orphaned muscle fiber. The other nerve (closer to the top of the illustration) still appears relatively healthy and functional.

The Recovery and Stable Stages

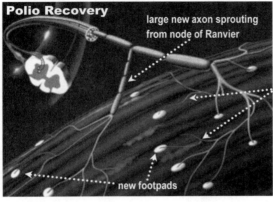

Figure 4: Reinnervation of the paralyzed muscle during the Recovery Stage.

As soon as the Acute Stage is over, the reinnervation of the Recovery Stage begins. Figure 4 reflects the successful reinnervation of the formerly paralyzed muscle. From the remaining healthy nerve (the upper nerve in the previous figures), several new axons, or nerve branches, have sprouted to replace the missing nerve. The larger axon sprout is originating from the area between two plaques of myelin. (This area between two plaques is called a *node of Ranvier* and is a common site for sprouting of new nerves to occur.) Axons also sprout from nerve branches and at the terminal portion of the nerve; examples of these can also be seen in Figure 4. Note that the footpads have regenerated as well. If you count the number of footpads and the number of new sprouts, you will see that the remaining nerve has had its workload and responsibilities more than doubled. Sometimes these surviving nerves will adopt many times the number of muscle fibers they were originally assigned.

It is only because many surviving nerves sprouted new axons, which then adopted orphaned muscle fibers, that some muscle function was reestablished after the acute polio infection.

I would remind you that axon sprouting is not unique to recovering polio survivors. Removal of decommissioned axons, and their consequent replacement by sprouting new axons, is a natural, ongoing, lifelong process in all of us. However, as a response to a viral infection, nerve regeneration by axon sprouting is unique to polio.[6]

Post-Polio Syndrome

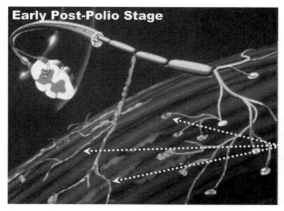

disintegration of axons that were regenerated after the polio infection

Figure 5: Disintegration of the regenerated axons.

---

[6] A possible exception to this statement has recently appeared: West Nile virus is capable of causing nerve damage similar to polio, and occasionally some nerve regeneration via axon sprouting appears in West Nile as well.

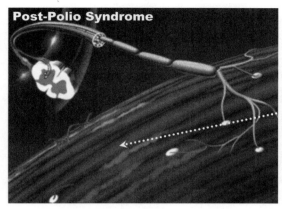

with degeneration of the axon sprouts that aided in the earlier recovery, the denervated muscle fibers result in reduced muscle function

Figure 6: Post-polio syndrome.

Figures 5 and 6 illustrate the deterioration that leads to post-polio syndrome. Observe the disintegration of the axon sprouts (which had developed during the Recovery Stage to adopt orphaned muscle fibers), leaving the muscle once again without a nerve supply. As noted above, nerve death followed by regeneration is a process that occurs normally and continually in all motor axons; however, in the case of nerves that matured from post-polio axon sprouts, there seems to be a premature (and probably an increased percentage of) replacement failure, resulting again in muscles without innervation. This second loss of innervation – this time without the nerve's ability to regenerate adequate replacement axons – eventually leads to a reduced functional neuromuscular mass. The weakness, pain, and tiredness associated with Post Polio come as a result of critically diminished neuromuscular mass.

It should be noted that some neuromuscular loss is normal as we age. It begins in early adulthood and is estimated by some experts to be about 1 percent per year. It increases considerably about the time we reach sixty, and the losses are cumulative – so all of our weakness as we age cannot be blamed on polio. However, if we as post-polio patients lose a motor nerve to this natural attrition, we may lose a nerve that services one thousand muscle fibers, rather than the one hundred fibers it was designed for, making our relative loss considerably greater than it would be in someone who never had polio. Remember, too, that we may have had many of our nerves destroyed at the time of our acute polio infection, leaving us with significantly fewer nerves to service our muscles. So, when one nerve in a polio survivor is lost to attrition, it is a greater portion of our total available nerves that is servicing a greater than normal volume of muscle fiber; therefore, it is easy to see that the normal *attrition of aging* has an exaggerated effect in Post Polio.

CHAPTER 3

VIRUSES AND POLIO: A PRIMER

The diagnosis of my polio made by the two young MDs in July of 1949 was a correct one. It was not necessarily a brilliant piece of medical detective work – polio was then in epidemic proportions throughout the United States, and its threat was ever present in the minds of physicians and parents alike. This chapter provides a primer on viruses in general and the polio virus in particular so that you can better understand the context of the epidemic of the mid-twentieth century in the United States.

The "Good Old Days" of Polio

Although polio was the most dreaded infectious disease in the first half of the twentieth century, it was not by any means new. An Egyptian stone carving of a priest dating back to circa 3000 BC showed atrophic changes in his legs, characteristic of polio. The way populations experienced polio five thousand (or even two hundred) years ago, however, was much different from ours in the twentieth century. The early- to mid-1900s was the first time that polio became global, afflicting massive numbers of people and resulting in a frightening amount of paralysis and death. Let me explain why.

Prior to the advent of modern hygiene systems, polio was a common intestinal (enteric) infection, passed from one person to another by fecal contamination. A person with an active polio infection produces billions of polio virus particles. Some of these particles are released into the tissues of the infected person's body, increasing the severity of his infection. The remaining particles, however, are released into his bowel where they mix with feces and are then discharged. One can see that with more primitive sanitation practices, essentially everyone was exposed to polio. This almost-universal exposure led to *community immunity*.

For example, if a mother had been infected with polio, she would then have immunity to that strain of polio virus and would pass that immunity to her baby in utero, providing a modest level of protection to the baby for six to twelve months. If the baby was then exposed to that strain during its first year of life, the mother's immunity would protect it from severe infection while it developed a permanent immunity of its own. At the same time, during the baby's infection, its fecal material would be washed away in the river where other members of the community bathed and washed clothes and dishes, infecting them with a low level of the polio virus against which they had developed a greater immunity.

So you see, essentially everyone was exposed to polio virus during childhood and developed some level of immunity. Therefore, even though *individuals* may have suffered from polio when they met with a strain of the virus to which they had insufficient immunity, there wasn't a large reservoir of non-immune people from which an *epidemic* might spring.

All that changed once modern hygiene practices were in play. When sewage no longer ran through the street and drinking water was piped and chlorinated, widespread exposure to the polio virus was reduced or eliminated. With reduced exposure to the virus, the immunity of entire communities waned, leaving large populations unprotected. Because the polio virus is highly contagious, these new, large, non-immune populations were easy prey. So, while improvements in hygiene markedly reduced many other infectious and toxic diseases, they actually facilitated the occurrence of polio in epidemic proportions.

The Polio Virus in the Twentieth Century

On the timeline of scientific discoveries, our understanding of viruses is very recent. We had our first glimpse of a virus only just over one hundred years ago. While performing experiments in the 1890s, scientists Dmitri Iwanowski and Martinus Beijerinck independently discovered that some material had slipped through newly developed filters designed to capture bacteria. At the time, bacteria were thought to be the smallest existing infectious agents, yet the infectious particles that passed through the filter were smaller. The newly discovered particles were given the name *virus*, derived from the Latin word for poison or toxin.[7]

It was also in the 1890s that the first polio epidemic in the United States occurred. In 1894, in Vermont, 132 cases of polio were reported, and with our improving public

---

[7] Nigel Dimmock, Andrew Easton and Keith Leppard, *Introduction to Modern Virology*, 6th ed. (Malden: Blackwell, 2007), 4.

sanitation, polio epidemics continued to crop up across the non-immune country.

In 1908, the polio virus was isolated for the first time, and polio became a reportable disease. Throughout the first half of the twentieth century, cases exploded at a rate exemplary of the full-on epidemic that it had become. Between 1945 and 1949, the United States averaged more than 20,000 new cases a year, and by the early 1950s, polio hysteria was in full swing. Meanwhile, the scientific world was in hyperdrive to find a vaccine to stop the epidemic. Growth of new cases had reached 58,000 in 1952 – a record year – and two years later (unfortunately, a little late for a lot of us) the polio vaccine was ready and initiated.

The results of the polio vaccine were nothing short of miraculous. By 1957, after a mass immunization campaign promoted by the March of Dimes, only about 5,600 cases of polio were reported in the United States, and in 1964, only 121.[8] In 1979, the last indigenous transmission of wild polio virus occurred in the United States. The research focus shifted as polio survivors began to experience similar symptoms decades after their recovery from polio. By the early 1980s, experts were congregating to discuss and evaluate these apparent late effects of poliomyelitis.

Before the polio vaccine, researchers had identified the polio virus by little more than its strains: Type 1, Type 2, and Type 3. Scientists noted that the types differed somewhat in potency and in the areas of the body that they preferred to infect, but that's about as much as was known. Today, we

---

[8] The March of Dimes was founded in 1938 as the National Foundation for Infantile Paralysis by President Franklin D. Roosevelt to defeat polio.

know how much the polio virus weighs, its size and dimensions, and its exact chemical composition. A team of Harvard scientists has even given us three-dimensional pictures of the polio virus, with and without its receptors.[9] The midcentury polio frenzy made polio the most studied virus in the world, and much of what we now know about virus infections in general was precipitated by this extensive research.

What the Polio Virus Is and Is Not

A *virus* is a completely inert, infectious agent made up of nucleic acid that is covered with a thin protein coating called a *capsid*.[10] We can't call a virus an *organism* because it has no organs; it has no metabolic apparatus that would allow it to move, grow, generate heat, or reproduce.

The polio virus is just a little thread of *ribonucleic acid* (RNA), wrapped in a capsid.[11] The RNA inside that polio capsid is similar to the gene material that is found in our

---

[9] In 1985, a team led by James Hogle of Harvard Medical School obtained high-resolution, 3-D images of the polio virus.

[10] The capsid is made up of plates (or subunits) called *capsomeres*. Depending on the arrangement of the capsomeres, which dictate the shape of the capsid, a virus is called an *isocohedral* or a *helical* virus. The polio virus is isocohedral. It has twenty triangular faces (capsomeres) and twelve corners. It reminds me of a Buckminster Fuller geodesic dome.

[11] The polio virus is a member of a group of viruses called *picornavirus*. The name comes from *pico* (meaning small), *rna* (referring to the single strand of gene material made of ribonucleic acid), and *virus* (the name originating from a Greek word meaning poison). From an infectious standpoint, it is important to know that polio is one of the smallest viruses. We will see how that works in its favor and to our detriment.

chromosomes – *deoxyribonucleic acid*, or DNA. Our DNA is a set of instructions to control and direct the activity and growth of whatever cell it inhabits. The RNA that makes up the polio virus is also a set of instructions – instructions on how to manufacture more of the polio virus. Unlike DNA, however, the RNA in the polio virus is without a cell to instruct. Before the polio virus can spread, it needs to find a way into a cell whose metabolic apparatus it can commandeer.

Like the contents of the envelope in *Mission Impossible*, the RNA contained inside the polio virus holds important instructions. These instructions must be delivered to a very specific site or they will be destroyed.

The Site of the Invasion: The Polio Virus Receptor

As an inert agent, the polio virus is unable to bore through the wall of the cell or actively invade it. For the polio virus to gain entrance, it must be received by the cell. This is done via a special receptor on the cell called a *polio virus receptor* (PVR), a secured entrance that says, "If you are a polio virus, I will receive you here."[12]

---

[12] The polio virus receptor was discovered by Columbia University graduate student Cathy Mendelsohn, PhD, working in the lab of Vincent Racaniello, PhD/MD. How real and how important is the PVR? In a well-documented experiment, Dr. Racaniello's laboratory team spliced a bit of human gene material that contained the human PVR into the gene sequence of a mouse. Ordinarily, the nervous system of a mouse cannot be infected with polio virus because it has no PVRs. However, after splicing the human PVR into the rodent's DNA sequence, the mouse became susceptible to all three forms of paralytic

An attachment must be formed between a matching receptor area on the polio virus and the PVR on the host cell, much like bringing together two pieces of a puzzle. Once the receptor area on the virus and the host cell's PVR are in proximity, tentacle-like threads of protein unfold from the virus, stabilizing contact while RNA is transferred from the viral capsid into the host cell.

It is important to note that every cell in our bodies contains a PVR. Most interesting to me is that the PVR is actually one of our genes – CD155. The CD155 gene is busily involved for the first four months of our embryonic existence with the development of the neuro-optical portion of our brain. Once that job is completed, the CD155 remains, but, apart from acting as the PVR, it is yet unknown whether CD155 serves any other function.

Having Its Way with Us: How Polio Multiplies

Being a bit of a romantic, I look at this transfer of RNA from the polio virus to the host cell as "the great deception," or as a "Trojan horse" phenomenon – naïve and foolish on the part of the invaded cell, for a couple of reasons. In the first place, the cell's PVR appears as a shamefully open invitation to the polio virus. Second, with the virus still on the doorstep, the host cell imprudently accepts the embrace of the virus's unfolded filament tentacles, paving the way for the transfer of

---

polio. This experiment not only proved a point, but led to the development of a strain of mice with the PVR. These mice have since been used to further polio research.

the deadly RNA.

I feel quite sure that the naïve host cell was unaware of what the virus had in mind. But like the Trojan horse, once inside the cell, the sweet-talking virus makes known its dastardly intentions, taking over the metabolism of the host cell and dedicating it to the manufacture of its own kind: the RNA instructions from the polio virus supersede the host cell's own set of instructions and redesign the cell to become a factory for the production of polio virus. The host cell's manufacture of the polio virus is intense and efficient. Shortly after invasion by the virus, the cell becomes so packed with virus particles that it ruptures, spewing out the newly manufactured virus and causing the dramatic death of the original host cell. (So much for romance at the cellular and sub-cellular level.)

Some of the spewed virus particles infect other host cells, leading to the manufacture of more virus and damage to more cells. The remaining virus particles spill into the bowel, contaminating the feces. This process will be repeated over and over until either the body's immune defense system has had time to build up enough antibodies to inhibit further infection, or the patient dies. In the meantime, the virus particles that were spilled into the stool are available to infect susceptible humans who might come in contact with it.

In most cases, the immune defenses work rapidly enough to avert a more severe infection, and the polio virus causes only low-grade, intestinal, flu-type symptoms in its victims. Sufferers may note fever, muscle aches, abdominal cramping, diarrhea, and fatigue, but may not even suspect polio.[13] Absent an adequate immune defense to the initial flu-type phase, however, the infection may spread from the intestine's lining cells into the bloodstream, infecting blood cells as well. This bloodstream infection is called *viremia*. The virus's reward for getting into the bloodstream is immediate dissemination to all areas of the body. Once viremia is in play, the potential for *paralytic polio* is born. Only one defensive barrier remains between the viremic stage and paralytic polio; this barrier is called the *blood-brain barrier*.

The Blood-Brain Barrier: The Last Line of Defense

The *blood-brain barrier* (BBB) is a physical and chemical barrier – a phenomenally complex network of tightly joined cells lining the inner walls of the blood vessels that approach and enter the brain and spinal cord. It prevents potentially harmful chemicals and parasites from leaking through the blood vessel walls into central nervous system tissues.[14] (In

---

[13] Less than 1%–2% of those infected suffer the paralytic and debilitating symptoms that we typically associate with polio. To distinguish this more severe form from the flu-type variant, it will be referred to as *paralytic polio*.

[14] The efficiency of the BBB sometimes works to our disadvantage. In addition to blocking deleterious parasites and chemicals from entry to the central nervous system, it also denies passage to certain therapeutic agents that might be used for treatment. By injecting an agent directly into the cerebrospinal fluid or by using massive quantities of it, the BBB can sometimes be bypassed or overwhelmed. Also, drugs are now being developed that use the BBB's active-transport systems to carry them through the barrier.

addition to serving as a barrier, the BBB has a second, and seemingly contradictory, function: through sophisticated, bi-directional transport systems, the BBB permits and actively promotes the passage to the central nervous system of certain hormones, nutrients, metabolites, and drugs essential to the healthy function of the brain and spinal cord.)

If the BBB is successful in keeping the polio virus from reaching the central nervous system, a polio infection is halted before it becomes paralytic. However, once polio virus penetrates the BBB, it can attack the nerve cells and with their destruction, paralysis will ensue. So: how can the polio virus get past the BBB?

Certain types of injury and inflammation can weaken the seal between the tissue cells that form the BBB, creating a defect that might allow virus particles or other foreign materials to pass into the central nervous system. Such is the case during the viremic stage of polio, when the quantity of virus infecting the blood and the associated inflammation are so great that fractures in the BBB may develop. Because the polio virus is so very small, it is able to gain access through these tiny defects. Once through the barrier, the polio virus attacks and destroys the cells of the central nervous system – transforming what might have otherwise been a relatively benign gastrointestinal infection into a paralytic form of polio.

Another method the polio virus might use to get past the BBB is one that the football enthusiast might call an "end run." During the viremic stage of polio when the virus has not yet penetrated the BBB, it has been shown that if the polio patient suffers damage to the blood vessels (e.g., a stab wound, abusive use of the muscles, blunt trauma), the virus may leak out of the broken blood vessels and attach to a polio virus receptor on a nerve in the area. The PVR would allow entrance of the virus to the nerve. The nerve then may carry the virus via its own transport system to its nucleus, where more virus is produced and the nerve cell is ultimately destroyed.

There is clinical support for this end-run theory in that many polio victims have reported that excessive exercise or trauma preceded their paralytic polio. President Roosevelt's polio history included excessive physical activity shortly preceding his paralysis. This possibility is especially interesting to me because in the week before my hospital admission, at which time I would have had viremia, I had been working in the July heat as an electrician's assistant. I spent much of my time in a hot attic, fishing wires through old walls. This involved kneeling, crawling, and lying on the two-by-four rafters for much of the day – an excellent way to traumatize the entirety of one's body. That trauma, coupled with the excessive heat, could well have been a factor in the severity of my disease.

It has also been shown that several individuals given injections (for any reason) shortly after receiving the Sabin polio vaccine developed paralytic-type polio in the area of the injection. As a result, those receiving the Sabin live-virus vaccine are now instructed not to have any other injections for a period of thirty days after receiving the oral vaccine to avoid having this occur.

A Bit about Vaccination

I feel certain that I am preaching to the choir here, but vaccination is so important that I will risk stating the obvious.

Vaccination to prevent polio is one of the most important things you can do for you and yours. Even if you have had polio, you could still have another infection of one of the two types that did not infect you the first time around. It is very important that everyone receive the recommended booster vaccinations. Remember, too, that it may take several weeks for your immune system to be adequately primed after a vaccination, so don't wait until it is time for you to go into an endemic area or until the epidemic is upon you to get your vaccinations and the recommended boosters.

There are two types of vaccine for polio: the *Salk vaccine*, which is made of dead, inactivated virus material, and the *Sabin (live-virus) vaccine*, which is made up of weakened polio virus that has lost its ability to infect and destroy the nervous system. The Salk vaccine contains antigenic material from all three types of polio virus. It activates memory lymphocyte growth and facilitates antibody production to all three strains.[15] The antibodies produced by the Salk vaccine will apprehend and destroy polio virus before it can invade the nervous system. It is a safe vaccine and cannot cause infection as it is made of inactive viral particles.

As a live-virus vaccine, the Sabin vaccine stimulates

---

[15] A memory lymphocyte is a type of white blood cell with a receptor on its surface that enables it to recognize a specific foreign substance. (See "The Immune Response: Mounting a Defense" in chapter 4.)

immunity by causing an actual polio infection using a weakened, non-paralyzing variant of the virus. Some feel the immunity produced by the live-virus vaccine is stronger and more permanent than the immunity produced by the Salk vaccine. Like the wild polio virus, the Sabin virus infects the bowel and when discharged becomes available to infect other people. In most cases, this is not a bad thing because infection with the weakened Sabin virus serves to extend the polio immunization program to people who would otherwise not have been vaccinated. There is a very small risk (less than one or two people in five million) that the Sabin vaccine can cause paralytic polio.

Some of the earlier concerns about each type of vaccine have been addressed by using a series of three of the Salk vaccine injections, or by using a combination of two injections of Salk and two doses of Sabin oral vaccine.

That a future mutation may produce a strain of polio virus resistant to existing vaccines is an ever-present possibility. To date, any mutational change in the virus has not been strong enough to start a new and distinct strain of polio. Current efforts at achieving universal vaccination and booster vaccinations are our best defense against a successful mutation in the future.

Postscript:
Moving Ahead with Polio Research

With our current understanding of how the polio virus is constructed, research is underway as to how the structure may be manipulated. In particular, two recent experiments have created excitement and some ethical controversy: one in the treatment of cancer, the other in the manufacture of virus by man.

Medical scientists at Duke University Hospital have excited the world by attaching anticancer drugs to a modified polio virus particle. The virus particle (with the attached anticancer drug) was then picked up by the patient's PVR and carried to the nucleus of the malignant brain cell – which it then destroyed. The malignant brain cells had retained their PVRs in exact enough form for the attachment of the cancer-killing polio virus to occur. Once this attachment was complete, the antitumor medications were carried into the cell (along with the polio virus), destroying the brain tumor cell, this time using the Trojan horse trick to the benefit of the patient. Turnabout is fair play.

In 2002, researchers at the State University of New York at Stony Brook inspired both excitement and controversy when they made polio virus from scratch. The researchers combined the chemicals that make up the polio virus in a beaker with a chemical cocktail similar to the primeval soup believed to have been present on the earth millions of years ago. In this milieu, the basic chemicals came together in the form of polio virus. The researchers then infected living tissues with the manmade virus, confirming its identity.

The ease with which the Stony Brook scientists were able to manufacture the polio virus raised fears that terrorists might replicate the process to create polio or other viruses known to infect and debilitate man. The manufacture of a virus also brought to the fore the question of whether a virus should be considered living matter or a simple chemical. Stony Brook University Professor Eckard Wimmer, in whose laboratory the polio virus was assembled, suggests that when the virus is outside of the cell it may be considered a simple chemical, but once inside, it functions as part of the cell and could be considered living material.

Though we have come a long way in our understanding and elimination of polio virus, it is still actively infecting many in other parts of the world. Likewise, there are still many unanswered questions surrounding Post Polio and post-polio syndrome. Our success in virtually eliminating polio in the United States over four decades ago means that the number of people afflicted by Post Polio here is probably reaching a peak at this time and will continue to dwindle in the coming decades until it dies out – as did polio itself. Nonetheless, it remains a fact of the future for the thousands and thousands of younger people around the world who suffered polio in the last forty years and therefore requires our continued study and attention.

CHAPTER 4

THE ACUTE STAGE: A FIGHT TO THE FINISH

Of the four stages of polio, the Acute Stage is clearly the most dramatic – essentially a fight to the finish between the polio virus and the body's immune system. It begins with the first exposure to the virus, and ends only when one side can declare victory. For those of us fortunate enough to have survived the Acute Stage, our immune systems ultimately prevailed; each of us, however, suffered our own battle injuries – some more serious than others. In this chapter, we will examine the war between our bodies and the polio virus to understand both the factors that influenced its outcome and the short- and long-term damage that it caused.[16]

---

[16] It should again be noted that, for the purposes of this book, I will primarily be discussing polio only in its paralytic form, the form in which the virus broke through the blood-brain barrier and infected the cells of the central nervous system, leaving the individual with loss of muscle function secondary to the destruction of his nerve supply.

The Pre-Clinical Phase: The Incubation Period

We can break the Acute Stage into two phases: the *pre-clinical phase* and the *clinical phase*. Pre-clinical is the very early phase of polio infection; it is the time when the number of virus particles and the amount of cell damage are very small. At this point, the battle between the body and the virus is invisible – the infected person cannot see or feel any symptoms and so has no idea that his body is under siege. The virus is engaged in a sneak attack.

This phase is also referred to as the *incubation period* and lasts roughly six to twenty days. During the later part, the polio virus is already being spilled into the feces of the infected individual, making him capable of spreading the virus to others even before he is aware of his infection.

I still don't know exactly how I picked up my polio virus. I come from a large family, and we were packed into our house like sardines, yet I was the only one who developed polio. At my summer job as an electrician's assistant, I was working pretty much alone, usually in remote areas, six days a week, so a work-related exposure seems very unlikely. On a few occasions during those weeks, a number of my friends and I snuck into a swimming pool that was under construction in our town. It was only partially filled with water, and I'm sure the purification system was not yet installed. I had not learned to swim, so I basically just floundered about and probably swallowed a good portion of the pool. That would seem a logical source of polio virus during a hot, Dakota summer. But again, I was the only one who developed the disease. So to this day the exact source of my polio remains a mystery.

From what we know about its incubation period, I can assume my first exposure to the polio virus occurred within a few weeks of my becoming noticeably sick in mid-July, 1949. As discussed in the previous chapter, the virus proliferates rapidly and efficiently, starting as soon as the first cell is infected. The infected cell then ruptures and pours out about a million viral particles, many of which infect more cells. The cycle of *host cell infection → replication of the virus in the host cell → rupture of the virus-packed cell → release of new virus, infecting more host cells → replication of the virus in the host cells* is repeated again and again, each time with more host cell destruction and an increasing virus population.[17]

The Clinical Phase: All-Out War

After a few generations of virus replication, the number of virus particles and dead host cell carcasses has increased markedly, and the presence of this increased amount of foreign material begins to be felt by the individual. Symptoms surface, marking the beginning of the clinical phase.

Initially, the clinical phase may manifest as merely a nonspecific sense of ill-being with sore throat and difficulty swallowing, progressing to include fever, chills, muscle achiness, headache, fatigue, and the like. As the clinical phase

---

[17] The total quantities of virus reach the billions. Remember, the polio virus has no way to propel itself and has to make contact with the polio virus receptor (PVR) of the host cell to commandeer the cell for virus-replication purposes. To do this, it must have those fantastically high numbers to ensure its future.

gains ground, vague muscle achiness subsides and localized pain increases in areas of the most severe underlying nerve destruction, ultimately resulting in weakness or paralysis of those areas.

According to the history the doctor obtained from my parents on the day I entered the hospital, I had not eaten well for the previous three or four days because of a sore throat and difficulty swallowing. These earliest symptoms marked the beginning of my clinical phase. I then developed the fever, chills, headache, and abdominal discomfort that caused my parents to seek medical help.

The fever and headache continued during the next four days and were joined by generalized muscle discomfort. By the end of that four-day period, my fever and nausea had subsided, but I was left with paralysis in my lower extremities. That was the extent of the Acute Stage of my polio. My polio infection was over.

The Immune Response: Mounting a Defense

Despite the havoc wreaked on our bodies by the invasion of the polio virus, most of us survived the Acute Stage. We were able to do this because our bodies have some pretty amazing defensive strategies and capabilities of their own, collectively comprising the *immune defense system*.[18]

---

[18] The immune response described here is composed of elements of both of our *innate immune system* and our *adaptive immune system*. Broadly speaking, the innate immune system is the "blunt instrument" that our bodies have at the ready to attack

The presence of foreign material in the body – bacteria, viruses, toxins, or anything else that is "not self" – sets off a series of immune reactions. These reactions begin with an *inflammatory response*, which may be experienced as swelling or achiness and fever. The function of inflammation is to increase the blood flow to the site of the invasion and to recruit and transport defensive cells, known as *immune cells*, that will help to fight off the foreign invader and, later, to repair the battle site.

The impressive defensive force includes a range of specialized immune cells, including cells that attack foreign invaders, cells that destroy host cells that have become infected or mutilated, cells that send out antibodies onto invaders to "mark" them for attack, and more. The virus is therefore greatly advantaged if it can achieve a deep and concentrated invasion during its sneak attack; once the immune system's highly skilled defensive army is activated, the invader is up against very significant odds.

Perhaps the most impressive aspect of the immune system in humans is the capacity to adapt its immune response uniquely to each new invader and to create an *immunological memory* that makes it impossible for the same invader to return and attack again. As you might have guessed, this is the basis for the effectiveness of vaccinations.

Let's look at this process in more detail as it relates to our polio infection.

---

whenever a foreign invader is detected; the adaptive immune system refers to those aspects of the process when the body is customizing the response to the polio virus specifically and creating immunity against future polio attacks.

The medical term *antigen* refers to any foreign substance within the body that triggers a reaction from the immune system. When someone is infected with the polio virus, the body recognizes as "foreign" not only the polio virus but also the dead host-cell fragments that remain after the rupture of those once-living cells. The body's goals are to rid itself of the viral antigen before the body is overwhelmed and to ensure that the virus is unable to attack again in the future. To achieve these goals, the enemy needs to be *recognized, cleared out,* and *put on record.*

The presence of antigens is first *recognized* by a group of ever-present proteins called the *complement system.* These complement proteins flow freely in the blood and can quickly reach the site of an invasion, where they make contact with the foreign intruders. This contact activates the complement system, which sounds the call to the immune defense.

In our bodies, we have eater cells known as *phagocytes,* which derive their name from the Greek words *phago* (to eat) and *cyte* (cell). Because phagocytes have an appetite for antigens, they are instrumental in ridding the body of foreign invaders. When the call is sounded, phagocytic white blood cells called *monocytes* are quick to respond. Monocytes pass through the blood vessel walls and into the threatened infected tissues. As a monocyte passes through the blood vessel wall, it transforms into another type of phagocyte known as a *macrophage* (literally, "big eater"). Once inside the infected tissues, macrophages engulf the polio virus and consume it, thus *clearing out* the enemy.

But the job of the macrophages in the immune defense

is twofold: in the process of consuming the polio virus particles, a part of the ingested virus (an *antigenic fragment*) is also taken to the surface of the macrophage for presentation to circulating lymphocytes. *Lymphocytes* are white blood cells that serve multiple important functions in our immune defense. On the surface of some lymphocytes – those known as *memory lymphocytes* – is a receptor that enables it to recognize a specific foreign substance.

Memory lymphocyte receptors are very specialized: each can match only one specific antigen. A memory lymphocyte travels through the body until it finds a macrophage that presents an antigenic fragment of the right size and shape to match its specific receptor. It might seem limiting that the receptor can only match one specific type of antigen, but the body produces such a large number of memory lymphocyte cells that there is a specific receptor for nearly any type of invader.

When the polio antigenic fragment presented on the macrophage's surface is recognized by a matching memory lymphocyte receptor, that memory lymphocyte is activated. At astronomical speed, the activated lymphocyte mass produces two types of immune cells: memory lymphocytes with polio-specific receptors identical to itself, and polio-specific, antibody-producing cells called *plasma cells*. The plasma cells turn out massive amounts of antibody. These antibodies from the plasma cells inactivate the polio virus and tag it for removal, and the memory lymphocytes *put it on record*.

Earlier, when I described the incubation period, I was describing the amount of time it took for the virus to multiply sufficiently and damage enough tissue to make us clinically aware of the infection. The body was scrambling to identify the invader as polio virus and then activate the appropriate lymphocyte to gear up antibody production to the level necessary to defeat it. If the person had had a previous infection with that polio virus or had been previously vaccinated with polio virus, the virus would have been on record, and there would have been a template team with many polio-specific memory lymphocytes already in place. Antibody production would have been on fast track with the ability to produce large amounts of antibody so quickly and efficiently that the infecting agent would not have been able to get a serious infection started. That is the beauty of memory lymphocytes.

The Inflammatory Response

Before we move on, I feel the inflammatory response deserves further mention, as it is such a key player in the body's immune defense. The entire cellular immune defense process is complemented and augmented by the inflammatory response that was set in motion when the complement proteins initially sounded the call.

If we were asked to define inflammation, most of us would be quick to list redness, heat, swelling, and possibly pain. And we'd be correct. However, there is much more going on with regard to inflammation. What we don't see or feel is the tremendously complex interactivity of mechanical, immunological, and chemical activities that are brought into play. The topic of inflammation is so robust that I will only skim its surface here, but let's look at how inflammation relates to our polio virus invasion.

I'll start with what can be observed. The *redness* that you see in inflammation is caused by the dilatation (enlargement) of capillaries and arterioles (little arteries) within the injured area of the body. Inflammation includes the same dilatation in internal tissues such as the heart, brain, and spinal cord, which we can't see or touch, as it does in more visible areas such as the skin, joints, and mucous membranes. Dilatation of these blood vessels allows more blood to flow to the site of the invasion. The blood carries the important cellular defense materials as well as oxygen, chemical enzymes, and various inflammatory proteins (cytokines) necessary for defense and healing. Dilatation of the blood vessels increases both the delivery speed and volume of these materials to the infected site.

The increased blood flow associated with inflammation also brings warm blood from deep within the body to the infected site, causing an increase in temperature. *Heat* not only speeds up the chemical reactions that put more defense elements into play, it also increases the permeability of the dilated blood vessel walls. Increased permeability allows enzyme-containing fluids to leak out of these dilated vessels and into the infected tissues. The additional fluid in the tissues results in *swelling*, which is beneficial in that it expands the work area so that the defense forces are better able to maneuver effectively within it.

In commercial media today, inflammation quite often gets a bum rap. It's seen as a symptom that needs to be alleviated – a part of the problem. But as you can see above, in our fight against the polio virus, inflammation is a vital part of the solution.

Factors Affecting the Battle

I have described the capabilities and tactics that each army automatically brings into the polio battle. However, for each case of polio, the way the battle plays out is unique, and a number of factors contribute to these unique outcomes.

One set of factors is related to the individual's *resistance*. The degree of tiredness, level of physical or mental stress, adequacy of nutrition and hydration, amount of disability from other disease, exposure to temperature extremes immediately prior to infection and during its active infectious stages – all of these factors and more may in some way affect the outcome of the disease. Avoidance of any of these would not have prevented the polio infection, but it may have played a very important role in the outcome of the battle.

Quantity of virus also plays a role in determining the severity of the disease. The larger the initial quantity of virus particles invading the body, the more host cells are commandeered and the more rapid and rampant the spread. A sudden, voluminous deluge of virus particles can overwhelm the body before the body's immune system has the chance to fully mobilize and produce an adequate defense, thus increasing the resulting severity of polio's destruction.

CHAPTER 5

THE RECOVERY STAGE: RETURNING TO OPTIMAL FUNCTION

The dictionary defines *recovery* as "to get back" or "to restore to the normal state." As polio survivors, we never did get back the full neuromuscular function that was ours before infection, and we never will be restored to a normal state. However, the degree of recovery we did achieve and the way we attained it are really somewhat miraculous. It can only be fully appreciated by those who have experienced paralysis, who had to be rolled from side to side in bed to prevent pressure sores, who needed to have an iron lung assist with their breathing, or who had to be lifted into a chair and fed by hand, and who now, by themselves, can turn over and climb out of bed, take a deep breath of fresh air without ventilator assist, or reach their mouth to feed themselves and brush their teeth. Whether recovery was obviously partial or apparently complete, coming as it did in the wake of the Acute Stage of our polio infection, the return of *any* degree of lost function felt like nothing short of a miracle.

The Recovery Stage began when the last of the polio virus infecting the nervous system was arrested and destroyed and ended months or years later when we "stabilized," having reached a point of maximal improvement. This chapter will address the symphony of processes that contributed to that recovery.

Reviewing My Own Chart

In working on this book, while sifting through memories of myself as a sixteen-year-old polio patient, I had a sudden inspiration. "There is no way …," I said to myself, "but I'll give it a try." With that, I dialed 411 and got the number for St. Luke's Hospital in Aberdeen, South Dakota. Upon reaching St. Luke's, I asked for Medical Records and then told a machine who I was and what I wanted. Fifteen minutes later, I got a call from a very pleasant lady named Karen, who sounded a bit excited and somewhat surprised at her own accomplishment.

"I was given your message and asked to look for your records," she said. "I have them all printed out for you!"

I sent the signed release form she requested, and in three days I had my hospital records from July through November of 1949!

Compared to today's stringent documentation requirements, medical records in those days were very brief, and mine were no exception. They did, however, correct, clarify, and confirm my recollections of the timeline of my hospitalization, including the dates that medications and therapies were started and stopped.

My memory, especially of the early days of my illness, is pretty sketchy. I recall the drive to the big city in the backseat of my brother-in-law's car, being swiftly admitted to St. Luke's, and waving good-bye to my sister Fran and her husband, Clarke, who were kept on the other side of a glass partition. As they wheeled me away, Fran appeared to be crying, which surprised me a bit because my sisters had always accused me of being spoiled ("spoiled rotten" I think was the actual term they used).

The nurses took all my clothes and dressed me in a hospital gown. They told me that the clothes I had worn to the hospital would have to be burned. (A second burning of all my possessions would take place a few weeks later when I was taken out of polio isolation and sent to the long-term care ward.)

The first night and the second day in the ward I was uncomfortable, but despite some headache, my mind seemed clear, and I communicated well with my roommate, the nuns, and the nursing staff. The hospital chart noted that, on the second morning, my legs were almost too weak to move and so weak that neither the strength in my legs nor the nursing staff would allow me to stand by the bedside without an attendant. Over the next two days, the weakness in my legs progressed. Although my arms and neck seemed a little weak, I could always move them, but after that second day, my legs were completely lifeless.

Treatments were started almost immediately and with intensity. I remember the hot packs, the muscle stretching, the exercises in the large Hubbard tub, and the electrical muscle stimulations that were administered those first three or four weeks. It was sometime in the third or early part of the fourth week that I noted some return of movement in my right great toe.

The toe movement was the first suggestion of recovery. Until that moment, despite coaxing by the physical therapist and all my grunting and pushing, trying and commanding, nothing had moved. So as soon as my toe movement was announced, I was surrounded by nurses, nuns, aides, and fellow patients who all wanted to see the movement. There was cheering and chanting: "Go, toe, go! Go, toe, go!" My exercise orderly looked on with obvious satisfaction; he was sure that this beginning recovery was all the result of his good work, and I certainly would not deny him a share of the credit. It was a great moment, but unfortunately for some of the latecomers, the toe muscle quickly fatigued and would no longer perform, bringing accusations of my making false claims and just trying to get attention.

Alas, the next day the toe movement returned for all to see. Again the nurses formed a cheering section. The naysayers accepted the undeniable and nodded approval. The nuns looking on smiled and then closed their eyes as they kissed their beads; they had their own idea about Who was responsible for my recovery. What a day!

As the days passed, the toe movement lasted longer, and soon I had added other movements to my repertoire. For the next few weeks, small but definite evidence of improvement was seen on nearly a daily basis. More muscles seemed to be awakening.

After the third or fourth week, I was able to perform more complex movements. My strength was improving too, albeit very slowly – too slowly for the likes of an impatient adolescent. The weeks ran into months. Antibiotics had been stopped by the end of the first month, as were the hot packs and the intense stretching sessions, which I had never liked. From then on, stretching was incorporated into my regular morning workout in the warm water of the Hubbard exercise tub. (Muscle and tendon stretching is much more pleasant after soaking in warm water for fifteen minutes!) After lunch and a rest period, I would have another session with physical therapy for strength building, more stretching, and, later on, gait training. These activities, tucked between periods of rest, filled my days.

By the end of the third month, I was learning to walk with crutches, and after a few weeks of practice, I earned my first weekend pass. It was fun to go home, but a lot more work than I ever expected. I couldn't wait to get back to the hospital, as I was exhausted. The second weekend pass was a bit better, but I still didn't resist returning to my bed in the hospital. My final pass came the day before Thanksgiving of 1949. That time I went home to stay, but I was not *recovered*. As I mentioned previously, it took me almost six years to reach what I felt was my point of maximum recovery. But I was home.

That briefly describes the beginning of the second stage of my polio experience – the Recovery Stage. Now, let's look at what took place in my body to bring about recovery.

Three Phases of the Recovery Stage

Recovery from paralytic polio is, at its heart, the result of nerve *axon sprouting* – the process whereby the surviving nerves sprout twig-like branches called *axon sprouts*. These axon sprouts grow down to and *reinnervate* muscle fibers whose original nerve supplies were destroyed during the acute polio infection, allowing these muscle fibers to function again. And, while the process of axon sprouting alone may qualify as the "polio miracle," the true genius of recovery also includes how the body prepared for that reinnervation and how it made use of those orphaned muscles once they had been adopted by a new nerve supply.

The Recovery Stage can therefore be divided into three phases: *cleanup, reinnervation,* and *optimization*:

- The *cleanup phase* involves cleaning up the battle site of the Acute Stage and restoring as much function as possible to the surviving tissues. This phase takes one or two months.
- As noted above, the *reinnervation phase* is the "big production number" of the Recovery Stage, and includes axon sprouting and growth – mind-bogglingly complex processes that result in a renewal of neuromuscular function following paralysis. Reinnervation takes approximately six months.
- During the *optimization phase*, three concurrent processes are at work to make the most of whatever neuromuscular function has been established via reinnervation. These processes – *hypertrophy*,

remodeling, and *accommodation* – will remain ongoing throughout our lives, but are significant in the Recovery Stage as they are the means by which the point of maximum recovery is reached. The length of this phase depends on a number of variables, including the severity and location of the original damage and the intensity of exercise and related efforts.

Let's look at how each of these three phases worked together to bring about our recovery.

The Cleanup Phase: Cleaning Up the Battlefield

The Recovery Stage technically began the moment the last virus was subdued. One could argue that the cleanup phase started even before the Acute Stage was complete. As explained in the last chapter, part of the immune response is to clear out not just the polio virus, but also the fragments of ruptured host cells that had fallen victim to the virus. So even before the Acute Stage was over, the macrophages were at the scene, encapsulating and digesting the dead and the debris.

The charge for the cleanup phase of Recovery is to get the house in order. Even in defeat, the polio virus has succeeded in leaving behind a landscape of devastation at the close of the Acute Stage. Dead cells and cell fragments, sick and injured cells, electrochemical imbalances, and excess fluids are all by-products of the Acute Stage. Before any serious axon (nerve) generation can take place, the mess must be cleaned up.

Rebalancing the Electrochemical Levels

If we were to look in on the involved tissues at the end of the Acute Stage, we would see that almost all of the nerve cells seem to be inactivated. The majority are ruptured and obviously dead. Some are injured but still intact enough to suggest that repair might be possible. And others appear well intact but with no function – not dead, but stunned.

To understand what is wrong with the cells that appear stunned but otherwise intact is important because, if we can resuscitate them, we could conceivably end up with a perfectly normal cell. In attempting to understand these stunned cells, you have to consider the chemical content of the fluid surrounding those cells (the "milieu," if you will). Recall that the body brought in additional fluid and chemicals as part of the inflammatory/immune response to the foreign invaders during the Acute Stage. While that fluid was critical to the defense system *during* the battle with the polio virus, the subsequent addition of leaked chemicals from damaged cells and vessels – including variable amounts of sodium, potassium, and calcium – can cause a serious disturbance in the electrochemical balance. Such *electrochemical imbalance* in the fluids bathing those cells can interfere with their circuitry and lead to the dysfunction that makes them appear stunned.

As the damaged cells' and blood vessels' walls are made

competent, that contaminated and excess fluid will be resorbed. When that is completed, the chemical levels in the cells and vessels can be returned to the levels needed for healthy function. The cells that appeared to be intact but stunned will begin to function again as the chemistry of the fluids around them returns to normal, and an adequate level of oxygen and nutrient supply is reestablished. Also, some of the injured cells will show some activity as evidence of mending. These first signs of cellular recovery take place in that first month.

The result of all of this is that, systemically, the infected person will begin to enjoy recovery as well because, as the toxicity of this electrochemically-imbalanced, post-inflammatory state is reduced, headache, fever, muscle pain, and other of the more overt symptoms of inflammation will begin to recede.

Following this symptomatic improvement will be signs of movement in some of the muscles that had been paralyzed. This is not yet due to the sprouting of new nerve axons but rather to the cleaning up of the war zone. Chemical imbalances produced by contaminated fluids simply shorted out the electrical circuitry of the nerve cells in the area, intoxicating and inactivating them, but not killing them. Once the debris is cleaned up, these cells begin to function again.

Those of us who aren't chemists have to be reminded that every chemical reaction is an electrical reaction of sorts. That's why we find positive charges on potassium and calcium and a negative charge on chloride, for example. These charges hold chemicals together to make compounds, or molecules. They also transmit signals from cell to cell. You can see how the changes of acidity, alkalinity, and temperature of fluids bathing the nerve cells might affect their function at the cellular level.

Removing the Dead Cells

As I've noted, one by-product of the Acute Stage is a lot of dead cells. If you are a tissue cell, you have two ways to check out or die: either by *necrosis* or *apoptosis*.

Very little of our polio cell death was by *necrosis*, which is ultimately due to loss of blood supply (often associated with trauma or vascular occlusive disease). Usually, when cells die a necrotic death, it is a group of cells rather than an individual cell. Dead cells that were once part of one's living body and are now inert debris are perceived by the body's defense system as foreign. As discussed in chapter 4, the body responds to foreign debris as an invader and sets up a defensive, inflammatory reaction. It will initiate the migration of macrophages to wall off groups of the virus and to ingest them or carry off debris. At the same time, lymphocytes and plasma cells are brought to the area to set up an immune defense. The inflammatory-type of response to foreign cells or tissue debris is usually associated with residual changes at the site, including scarring and deformity, which, for reasons I'll discuss later, will prevent any significant reinnervation of the muscles.

Fortunately for our recovery prospects, most cell death from polio was by *apoptosis*. Apoptosis is fascinating, and very different from necrosis. With apoptosis, there is a dismantling of the nonfunctioning cell. A group of enzymes called *capsases* come in and cleave the cell at very specific points so that the cell is broken into pieces that the body can use. Then a membrane forms around the cleaved pieces, which essentially "packages" them. The packaged material is ingested by macrophages and then made available to cells throughout the body. It is kind of like a "chop shop," where thieves disassemble stolen cars and sell the parts, rather than smash them whole for scrap metal. It appears that because the membrane-packaged fragments are analogous to "approved, factory-made parts," they are not considered foreign by the immune system and therefore do not trigger an inflammatory or immune reaction. With no inflammatory activity, there is no scarring or damage to adjacent tissues and blood supply. This is important for a couple of reasons.

First, the tubular endoneural sheaths that surrounded the nerve fibers are left intact. A new axon sprout cannot grow to an orphaned muscle fiber unless it has an old endoneural sheath to grow through, direct it, and nourish it along its way.

Second, because it reduces the collateral loss or damage to adjacent nerve and glial tissues that accompany necrotic disruption of blood and nutrient supply, it makes apoptotic nerve loss very discreet. It can remove a single dysfunctional nerve without adversely affecting those around it, as if it were whisked away in the middle of the night.

Polio had to have worked out a deal with our bodies

because it is clear that the polio virus induces cell death via apoptosis, and we could not have survived central nervous system polio without it. Our parasites need us for their species' survival. Because we are polio's only host, if each person infected with polio died, polio would die out as well.

The Reinnervation Phase: Giving Orphaned Muscles a Second Chance

Once the cleanup is over and the electrochemical imbalances, excess fluids, dead cells, and other detritus are no longer stealing the spotlight, the stage is set for Recovery's big act: reinnervation.

As you'll remember from the illustrations in chapter 2, some motor nerves were casualties of the battle of the Acute Stage, leaving their associated muscle fibers without a source of movement impulse from the brain. During the reinnervation phase of Recovery, the remaining functioning nerves actually sprout new *axons*, which grow and endeavor to connect with the orphaned muscle fibers to enable them to move again.

As a new axon sprouts, the tip, called the *growth cone*, begins to grow; the growth cone acts as a feeler, searching for an intact *endoneural tube*. As noted earlier, thanks to previous nerve cells' apoptotic deaths, finding an abandoned but useable endoneural tube is an achievable goal for the new sprout. Once the growth cone has found one, it will lead the axon sprout down the endoneural tube where (if all goes well) the axon will proceed at the rate of 1–4 millimeters a day to reach an orphaned muscle fiber. If it cannot make appropriate contact, the axon will wither away.

A motor nerve axon is extremely thin and long; its length may be 1,000 to 10,000 times the diameter of its cell body, all in one strand, reaching from its cell of origin in the spinal cord to its destination (the muscle in a toe or calf, for example).

Various growth factors and attractants participate in the delivery of an axon to an orphaned muscle fiber. Schwann cells on, and other glial cells in, the wall of the endoneural tube facilitate axon growth by producing growth-stimulating factors and providing nutrition for the nerve sprout along its way.[19] (The axon sprout needs the endoneural tube not only for the period of axon regrowth but for lifetime maintenance of the nerve fiber). Direction and growth are also encouraged by signals from N-CAM (Nerve Cell Adhesion Molecule), a material that collects on the surface of the denervated but viable muscle fiber. N-CAM appears to act as an attractant and a target for the axon, attracting the axon to its site and then participating in its signal-receiving contact with the muscle fiber.

---

[19] The glial cells and Schwann cells are part of a massive support system for the nerves. The glial cells, which outnumber nerve cells about 9:1, supply the nerves with nutrients and oxygen, have primary responsibility for maintaining the electrochemical balance in the brain and the spinal cord, and help deter pathogens. The glial support system also provides structural support and protection to the nerve tissues, largely in the form of myelin insulation sheathing that covers the nerve axons and surrounds the sites where the nerves connect (synapse) with the muscle or with other nerves. One of the Schwann cells' major functions is to wrap the myelin around the nerves. This endoneural sheath both physically protects the nerve fiber and increases the speed and the privacy of the messages transmitted along the nerve.

Initially, regenerated axons are thin and non-myelinated (noninsulated), so their conduction velocity is very slow. With time, the Schwann cells will insulate these fibers with myelin, which will speed up their conduction and hopefully return it to near normal.

Although beautifully complex, this process is not always perfect. For example, sometimes the newly sprouted axon ends up reinnervating a different type of muscle fiber than that for which the "parent" nerve was designed, so the muscle has to be modified so that it can function in accordance with its new nerve supply. For example, if the nerve axon sprout is from a nerve associated with endurance-type muscles (Type I muscle fiber – found in our postural muscles and those needed for long-distance running), and it ends up climbing into and growing down an abandoned endoneural tube associated with an activity-type muscle (Type IIa or IIb muscle fiber – found in the muscles we use for swimming or sprinting, for example), the Type II muscle fiber must be modified chemically and anatomically to function as Type I fiber. This will take time. Sometimes the footplate is not completely functional, so it can't release the chemical signal to the muscle receptor. Sometimes the nerve cell's metabolic system cannot adequately support the new axon sprouts because of overload – simply too many axons or too long a distance. Many axons may sprout from parent nerve cells that suffered damage and therefore may not be able to function optimally when stressed. These less-than-perfect reinnervations may also make these nerves more subject to early death.

Optimization: Maximizing Our Recovery

The cleanup phase was completed in the first month or two after our infection. That cleared the way for reinnervation via axon sprouting, which started in earnest after cleanup and was mostly completed in the next six months. We felt better by this time, but certainly weren't recovered. Many of us felt it took five or six years to reach our point of maximal improvement. Just getting well after an overwhelming infection associated with a long period of inactivity takes time, but we needed more than just a period of rest to accommodate the damage to our bodies and souls caused by the polio virus. We needed time to incorporate and learn to make the most of whatever function we'd been made capable of through the reinnervation process.

Fortunately, our bodies were fully aware of that need and already implementing three new programs to augment the benefits of viral eradication and muscle reinnervation: (1) muscle hypertrophy to improve strength, (2) tissue and structural remodeling to make better use of viable tissues that remained, and (3) lifestyle accommodations to survive, live comfortably, be productive, and be accepting of post-polio deficiencies. These programs were critical in achieving the point of maximum recovery, and they will continue to play an important role throughout the polio survivor's life.

Building Muscle Size and Strength

Once the reinnervation of polio-orphaned muscle fibers is complete, increasing strength can begin. About the only way to increase strength is to hypertrophy the remaining muscle. *Hypertrophy* means enlargement, and in this case, it refers to enlarging the muscle fiber by increasing its content of contractile proteins: *actin* and *myosin*.

The amount of contractile proteins in post-polio muscles varies with exercise and will diminish with disuse and rebuild with activity. Hypertrophy of residual muscle is a dynamic compensatory process, compensating for the numbers of lost muscle by increasing the strength and size of remaining muscle. As with normal muscle, appropriate exercise is necessary to maintain it and to get maximum performance from it.[20]

Remodeling

Architects and interior decorators use the term *remodeling* to conjure up images of fresh beauty, improved function, and better ideas. In medicine, however, remodeling relates to the tissue modifications that the body makes to preserve a degree of function in an area that has suffered loss. Rather than a permanent fix or a better idea, remodeling in the medical sense is more often a stop-gap rearrangement that, with time, will prove inadequate and have to be further reinforced. Remodeling with regard to polio is different for every survivor. The polio infection impacted each of us uniquely, in terms of degree and the areas affected. The remodeling the body does is very specific to one's defect.

---

[20] In extreme cases, hypertrophy might be too much of a good thing. If muscle fibers get too big, the ability to get adequate nutrition and nerve impulse stimulation to their depths may be impaired, resulting in loss of force and speed relative to their excessive increase in size.

Take my polio-weakened left leg as an example. If we had studied my knee at the time I broke my leg, we would have found that the support muscle around the knee was very thin; in its place was a lot of scar tissue intermingled with strands of dark red muscle tissue. The tendon and fibrous connective tissue that make up the joint capsule had become significantly thickened in their attempt to stabilize the joint, but by this time, they were badly stretched, allowing my knee joint to be a bit loose and for my knee to bend back. We would have seen that the knee-joint stress caused by the recurvatum had resulted in loss of cartilage and erosion of the joint surface, a picture consistent with degenerative (traumatic) arthritis.

It wasn't perfect, yet my body's remodeling of that extremity allowed me to function effectively and without significant discomfort for a long period of time, even though the correction was not as good as new. The few muscle fibers that were left hypertrophied, which gave them greater strength. The darkness of the muscle fibers suggests that they had been switched to Type I, fatigue-resistant fibers, which would increase endurance. The thickening of scar tissue was my body's further attempt to stabilize the joint. However, over time, the abnormal strains and pressures interfered with the blood flow and nutrition of the joint, which led to loss of cartilage and production of small ulcerations in the joint surface.

For several decades after my acute polio infection, I had no significant pain. But now – with an abnormal strain of recurvatum, bone rubbing on bone (resulting from loss of joint cartilage), arthritic pitting of the joint surface, and progression of weakness due to decreased muscle mass – I am more than likely to have pain.

Often, the failure of a remodel is partly the survivor's fault, as he has misused or abused the remodel in one way or another. He has gained weight, failed to exercise, refused to use a brace, or unnecessarily put himself in harm's way. I did it. That was my knee we were just talking about, and I did abuse it. I gained a bit of weight, I waited far too long before using a brace, and then, by trying to get somewhere without my walking stick, I put myself in harm's way and fell and broke my leg.

Accommodation

As its name implies, the accommodation process involves all of the adjustments we make to accommodate our disability, allowing the whole body and mind to accept and live productively with the various changes resulting from the polio infection. Consciously or subconsciously, we make the decisions on how to accommodate or adapt to the postinfectious residual on the basis of intelligence, motivation, desire, interests, level of emotional and physical discomfort, environment, social situation, and so on. This is our call.

For me, the choices I made turned out pretty well. I married the right woman, and we, fortunately, got the right kids. Our climate allows me to get around throughout the whole year, albeit with some limitations. I cannot climb ladders, so it's good that I didn't become an electrician. I couldn't stand around the operating table for six or eight hours at a spell, so I'm much better off as an internist than as a surgeon. The majority of the decisions I made were good. They allowed me to enjoy a pleasant, rewarding, and productive life.

The "end" of the Recovery Stage is not likely something the polio survivor celebrated with balloons and cake or a glass of champagne. Instead, it probably snuck up on him, and he didn't realize it had happened until he was able to see it in the rearview mirror. The Recovery Stage came to an end when the body and mind had done all that was possible to maximize improvement and optimize quality of life following the polio infection.

CHAPTER 6

THE STABLE STAGE: APPARENT STASIS

The Stable Stage is how I refer to the period between the point of maximum recovery and the point at which we have accumulated sufficient symptoms (increasing weakness, easy fatigue, pain, etc.) that our post-polio impacts are influencing daily life.

"Stable Stage" is a misnomer in two ways. First, it is not truly stable, as during this period we polio survivors were indeed experiencing the same physical impacts of aging that all humans do – an ongoing, and decidedly unstable, process. And, second, it is a "stage" only by default – an intervening period between two other stages.

To better understand the Stable Stage, let's zero in first on the starting point: our functional capabilities and neuro-muscular reserves at the point of maximum recovery and how they compared to those of our non-polio peers.

Then, we'll explore the *natural attrition of aging* and see how this universal process can have a seemingly amplified effect on those of us who have survived a polio infection – and may lead to the collection of symptoms that define Post Polio.

Function and Reserves at the Point of Maximum Recovery

I noted in chapter 1 that I felt I'd reached my point of maximum recovery about six years after my acute polio infection. I was beginning medical school, had boundless energy, and felt no conscious need to accommodate my polio. Does that mean that my physical functions and capabilities were exactly what they would have been if I hadn't had polio? Of course not. Does it mean that they were exactly the same as every other polio survivor's? Again, of course not.

Though I reached a point where I felt that, from a social, professional, and family standpoint, my life was not much different from those of my non-polio friends, polio had left its marks on me.

The marks that polio leaves are different for each survivor. Although my infection primarily affected my legs, I spent much of my so-called "stable period" walking unaided, and many people didn't notice anything unusual in my gait if they didn't look too closely. On the other hand, I never went up a flight of stairs without making significant use of the handrails, I never golfed or jogged or played tag or football. It became second nature for my kids to pause in front of me as they stepped off a curb to cross a street so that I could put my hand on their shoulder to balance as I stepped down.[21]

---

[21] My wife and I had five beautiful, active children who kept us busy. Although I was not able to run, play ball, or climb trees with them, I compensated in other ways, and they feel I did a good job of parenting. They sometimes found an advantage in my inability to run, jump, or climb. When they got me upset and I started after them, shouting orders, they would run for

Many polio survivors came through the Recovery Stage with much more obvious impacts than mine, and many with much less so. Each of us had our own unique set of residual effects – some so subtle as to be virtually unnoticeable, and others nearly impossible to ignore. In nearly every case, however, we can be confident that the polio infection left us with less than we'd had before waging war with it. One element of our loss was the reduction of our *functional neuromuscular reserves*. Let me explain.

Human beings are blessed with a tremendous amount of reserve. We are born with about twice as much of everything as we need. We can get along nicely with one good kidney, one good gonad, one good lung, or one-half of our thyroid – and we could function at a normal level with the equivalent of 50 percent of our birth-given *functional neuromuscular mass*. Neuromuscular mass refers to muscle fibers innervated by motor nerves; innervation renders the muscles functional. So if we start out with twice as much functional neuromuscular mass as we need, our functional neuromuscular reserves are the second half of that mass.

For example, if, at the time of acute polio infection, you experienced total paralysis in the lower extremities and generalized weakness elsewhere, you may have lost 85 to 90 percent of your motor nerves and associated muscle function. If axon

---

the stairway, get halfway up the stairs, then stop, turn around, and grin, "How far are you going to count this time, Dad – to three or to ten?" They knew full well that I could not catch them on the stairs. I continue to be their straight man or the fall guy for their jokes. They all turned out quite well. They give me some credit for that, but to give credit where credit is due, they had a fantastic mother.

sprouting reinnervated half of the muscles, you might have the equivalent of about 55 percent of your pre-infection functional neuromuscular mass. For a moment, that sounds very good – I've already said you should be able to function very effectively with half of your original neuromuscular mass. But if you end up with 55 percent of your pre-polio neuromuscular mass at the point of maximum recovery, that means that you have lost nearly *all* of your *reserves* to the polio infection.

As a Depression baby in South Dakota, I grew up with a constant concern, conscious or subconscious, about reserves (or, more accurately, the lack thereof). Those reserves, of course, were of the material kind. I started many a trip with four semi-bald tires and a spare that had been patched time and time again; and I can remember my mother sewing a dollar bill into my shirt pocket so that I would have some money in reserve should I need it. Reserves, during the Depression in South Dakota, were not a plentiful item. Many of us were living on the brink.

One Saturday morning, when I was in medical school, I asked my wife for some money to service the car. I explained to her that we were out of gas and that we needed oil as well. After a somewhat emotional lecture on the status of our finances, she very reluctantly gave me two dollars, in dimes, nickels, and quarters, and told me to go ahead with the purchase of gas, but "don't waste money on oil." The phrase "don't waste money on oil" has since been a family joke.

At the end of the Recovery Stage, we polio survivors felt we were "healed." We were doing well. Why should we need more? When we reached that point in our recovery, we were jubilant. Some of us appeared nearly indistinguishable from our non-polio peers; others of us had made peace with polio's visible impacts. Given that we could function quite adequately, we very possibly gave no thought to the fact that we might be traveling without a spare. Unfortunately, despite its name, the Stable Stage is a time of life when polio and non-polio folks alike start to rely on their "spare."

Natural Attrition of the Aging Process

Medically, we use the word *attrition* to refer to loss of strength, function, or capacity as a result of aging and wear. Physical medicine experts tell us that adults lose about 1 percent of their neuromuscular function per year, with the total loss of neuromuscular mass reaching approximately 50 percent by eighty years of age.[22] This is something that happens to all of us and is referred to as the *natural attrition of age*. For someone with a normal amount of muscle, it takes a long time for this loss to be noticeable. Most professional football, hockey, or basketball players feel that they are over-the-hill due to neuromuscular attrition by thirty-five to forty years of age. But for someone not pushing his muscles to function at that high level of performance, the loss may not be noticed until he reaches the mid-forties, even later if he has maintained a good general exercise program through regular workouts, work, and the activities of daily living.

---

[22] It is interesting that with this process of aging we also lose the muscle-type balance that we had when younger, losing a larger percentage of the muscle fibers that allow for quick-response movements and ending up with a predominance of the fibers recognized for greater endurance but less strength.

Those of us with polio undergo the same natural attrition of aging as those without polio, only when we lose 1 percent of our original (pre-polio) neuromuscular function, we lose a much greater proportion of our current function. We may have already lost 40 to 90 percent of the nerve supply to our muscles as a result of our acute polio infection, so our attrition must come out of that residual neuromuscular mass. Also, because of axon sprouting, the neuromuscular unit we lose through attrition may be serving two to twenty times more muscle fibers than the neuromuscular unit of a person without polio. With this understanding, we can see why our loss of strength with aging may progress more rapidly than that of our non-polio peers and why many aspects of Post Polio might be caused by attrition associated with aging.

In all of us, throughout life, a number of our nerve axon branches deteriorate and are replaced by new axon sprouts, whether we have had polio or not. This appears to start out as a fairly balanced process, occurring on a regular basis, with each axon sprout that becomes dysfunctional being replaced by a new one. We have assumed that that is the way it was meant to be. And if it had continued to work that way, the Stable Stage would have been a "stable" period. But it doesn't work that way, for us, or for our non-polio peers. Regeneration or replacement does not keep up as we age; hence our non-polio peers end up with loss of about 50 percent of their birth-given neuromuscular mass by age eighty, and we end up with Post Polio – most often long before we become octogenarians.

CHAPTER 7

OBSERVING THE BATTLE: A FICTIONAL REVIEW

Let's have a little fun reviewing what we've learned so far about how the polio virus attacks the body and how the body responds.

Imagine that several of us have been sent in as an observation team to evaluate the attack that the Polio Virus launched on the Body. At this time, the acute phase of the war is over, and recovery is underway. As observers, our emphasis will be on the Central Nervous System (CNS) front, where we are to assess the amount of destruction, analyze the reparations already underway, and estimate the degree of recovery we might expect.

At this point, although enemy troops have been essentially eliminated from the CNS, there is the possibility that a small but significant number are still hiding out on the Gastrointestinal (GI) front. These troops may continue trying to escape from the Body for another two to ten weeks and, if successful, invade another Body to wage another war. We feel lucky that if any remaining sniper activity is to occur in this Body, it will probably be on the GI front, rather than on the CNS front, which we are being asked to observe. As official observers, we have been briefed on what to expect in the way of inflammation, attrition, necrosis, and apoptosis. Yes, we feel rather comfortable with our level of intellectual preparedness.

We have been impressively equipped with specially designed coveralls with attached hoods and gloves made of a new lightweight material designed to resist water, float, and tolerate environmental heat up to 105º F. The lightweight, waterproof boots have a slip-resistant sole that is amazingly effective. Our protective glasses have normal and infrared lenses with up to 100× magnification. These outfits sound a little ducky, but we actually look really sharp. Cameras are not allowed, for fear of setting off a methane explosion. We have been advised to observe carefully and to carry the images in our heads so that we can brief Headquarters when we return.

Our Guide starts us off with a surprise: because repair work is being done high in the Nasopharynx, we will not be able to enter the CNS via a known fracture in the Blood-Brain Barrier (BBB). That is unfortunate because our Guide is very familiar with the Nasopharynx and Tonsil regions – having scouted those areas as a spy during the initial invasion – and he had actually seen a fracture in the BBB where he thought we should enter. Instead, we will have to enter via Anal Pass, potentially exposing us to enemies that could be hiding in the crypts of the GI terrain. The Guide apologizes and offers to excuse any of us who feel the risk is more than we want to take. Fortunately, everyone decides to stay on, which is nice because we have started to feel like a team.

They have already reprogrammed the Miniaturizing

Chamber at the newly appointed site for our entrance to the Body. The six of us enter the chamber, one at a time, and are reduced in size so that we can travel very comfortably in the area we have been assigned to observe.

Our entrance via Anal Pass is uneventful. We are amazed that the landscape is as well healed as it is. There are some patches of redness and some watery engorgement of a number of the villi, reminding us that part of the war had been fought here. Villi are tall, frond-like projections that, we were told, make up much of the terrain in this area. We measure the depth of the crypts between the villi; in some areas, they are very deep. You can see how the enemy might be able to hide and survive in this GI area for days, or even months, after the war in the CNS was won.

About the time we are celebrating the fact that we have not seen any enemy troops, the Guide tells us to try using the 100× magnification on our glasses and look carefully in almost any direction. With that, the picture changes. With magnification, we see a number of enemy troops peeking out of crypts and a few sneaking out of their hiding places and climbing into waste material that the Body was preparing to export. At this point, that is about the only way they are going to get out of the Body intact. A couple in our group want to go after them, but the Guide reminds us that we are here to observe and report, not to fight.

We continue to climb for a rather long distance. We notice a change in terrain as the villi begin to vary in size and shape. The Guide tells us that he can deduce what area of the GI front we are in by the shape and size of the villi. We can see several areas that had been rather badly torn by the war, but most of the damage caused by the enemy appears to be pretty well healed over by this time. We gather in one area to explore the repair process more closely.

The Guide decides that this is a good place and time to give us more history of the war to prepare us for the next step in our journey. He tells us that about three weeks ago he had been working as a spy for the Body and was hiding and observing from a place high in the Nasopharynx, just above the Tonsils, at the time the enemy invaded. He said that the enemy's troops entered in such massive numbers that, although the Body was in good condition, it was obvious that the Body's natural resistance measures might not hold the enemy at bay long enough to get Immunity involved in the early battle. He could see that it was going to be a vicious fight and that, even if the Body did survive, there would be lots of life lost.

Shortly after the invasion started, the Guide had to change his observation hideout. Apparently, the enemy troops overwhelmed the defensive troops in the Nasopharynx and Tonsils on their way in and were causing severe damage. The Guide said he slipped away to distance himself from the fighting and find a place where he could more objectively observe the conflict. The spot he chose was only a few paces from where we are now sitting.

It was obvious at the outset that the enemy knew exactly what it wanted, and wasted no time getting it. The number of the enemy's troops was such that the Body's GI Lining Division, which would ordinarily serve as its first line of defense, was devastated in the first round or two.

"Instead of killing our troops outright," the Guide said, "the enemy overpowered the Body's troops in the GI Lining Division and forced each of them to manufacture about one million new enemy troops."

So as the Body's troops fell, the enemy troops actually increased in number, at least during the early part of the conflict. The Guide told us that, if the Body's troops did not die in that process, they were left to die.

The Guide becomes a bit misty as he remembers the once-proud GI Lining Division cells who had been forced to produce enemy troops. It was such a humiliation, having to give your life and, while still in the process of dying, being aware that you are aiding the enemy in doing harm to your still-living comrades. The enemy obviously paid no attention to the Geneva Accord.

Several of us ask why the war zone looks so good if the invasion was so massive and loss of life so enormous. The Guide tells us that the normal cell lifespan was short in the GI region and in Blood. He explains that when the enemy troops destroyed one of the Body's GI or Blood troops, a new unit was already lined up to replace it in a matter of hours or days, hence the neatness – the almost-healed GI front – only two or three weeks after the invasion. He said that we would find things much different on the Central Nervous System battlefield because the lifespan of cells from that area is usually more or less the length of the Body's life. In the CNS, there are no new bodies standing in line to replace the dead – a life lost is irreplaceable and scars are permanent. We are beginning to get the picture.

With that, the Guide looks at his watch and frowns. He had noted earlier that there was a vessel belonging to Blood located just below us. The Guide decides that, since time is getting short, we should enter the vessel and then let Blood's current carry us to a large fracture in the Blood-Brain Barrier that the enemy had used during its CNS invasion. The Guide had used it several times before while spying and, provided it has not been repaired, is sure we will have no difficulty squeezing through, saving us time and distance.

Fractures in the BBB are quite rare and are not seen except as a result of the ravages of war or other severe trauma. Here, the enemy had hit so quickly and with such an enormous number of troops that, after the second or third offensive battles, they had literally swarmed through the defense on the GI front. They had then established themselves solidly into Blood, whose tubular infrastructure gave them access to almost every part of the Body.

The Guide reminds us that, at the time of the initial invasion, the Inflammation Division, with its Necrosis Unit, is still about the only defense the Body has available. And even though Inflammation could damage the BBB, allow the enemy access to CNS, and (with its attendant necrosis and scarring) would itself cause some irreparable damage to CNS, its methods had to be excused because, until Immunity's forces could be adequately mobilized, Inflammation was the only means the Body had of confronting the enemy.

The Guide won't tell us more. He simply says we'll see for ourselves shortly. We can see from the look on his face that his emotions will not let him continue. He changes the subject and soon finds one of Blood's channels for us to enter.

Blood's hydraulic transfer system is nice. Getting the weight off our feet for a while feels marvelous, as does the warmth. We cannot talk, so we communicate with an occasional wave or a smile and once in a while point to something of interest. It is a good trip, and we all wish it could last a bit longer.

We help each other climb out of Blood's vessel and through the crack in the BBB. Once on the other side, we are able to look out onto the Central Nervous System battle site. The different emotions we experience in those first seconds are too numerous to count. Such devastation. Such waste. I feel an anger build up in me. But as I continue to take in this horrific battle site, I am overcome with a deep appreciation for the gift of vaccination. I could not understand how anyone could be against Immunity's desire to see that everyone on this planet is supplied with a few antibody troops and a personal template to protect against this type of devastation. The special glasses we are wearing hide the many tears being shed by our group this day.

The Guide, who earlier had trouble bridling his own emotions, brings us up abruptly by reminding us of the hour and the size of our task. Before we scatter to study the site, though, he wants to apologize if he has given the impression that the Body's defense was loose, lazy, or slow to respond. He explains that, at times, it looked that way because of the massive numbers of the enemy, but that he had seen the Macrophage troops responding from the start, and Immunity's

Template Division troops had been right there with them. Immunity's handling of the whole war had been unbelievable. By getting its Lymphocytes and Plasma Cell troops into the fray at the first sign of invasion, it had been possible to get a template enabled and distributed for use. With the template available, Immunity was able to produce enough antibody troops to come back and defeat the enemy. The Guide assures us that, until the very last minute, a gambling man would never have bet on the Body, but the Body's troops came through.

I am most surprised by the Glia. Most of us have never heard of them. Now, inside the BBB, we are seeing evidence of them all over the place. The Guide tells us that Glia has a payroll nine times the size of the CNS's and that Glia is almost totally responsible for the maintenance and the structural support of the CNS. Glia supplies the necessary blood, nutrients, chemicals and growth hormones, so that the CNS can go about its important business of creating, sending, and receiving messages. He tells us that Glia screens almost all of the CNS's messages and directives and will, if it deems it necessary, modify some of them. (On rare occasions, Glia may even initiate and send messages of its own.)

Looking down on the battlefield, we can see where various Macrophage troops have moved in to wall off and neutralize the invader. As phagocytic cells, Macrophages are "eaters" and are busy on an everyday basis, engulfing, transporting, and digesting dead and foreign material such as inactivated viral particles, tissue fragments, and the like. They excel when the enemy is Bacteria. The Guide tells us, however, that in a battle with the likes of our Enemy (polio virus), the Macrophages show industry and versatility above and beyond the everyday. In the heat of battle, some Macrophages will actually aid the Immunity Division by serving as Immune troops. As the Guide looks out at the Macrophages at work, he explains that they only work for about a month and then they're gone, so none of the workers below are familiar to him. (We did not find out until later that they work until they die, which is why none of the old crew was still around.)

We could see Lymphocyte and Plasma Cell troops that had been moved into this area to initiate more immune defense activity. The Guide, who spied on this area at the beginning of the war, seems to recognize a few of them as having been there from the start. Genetically, Lymphocytes belong to the Memory Division and are blessed with a fairly long life. That's the reason Immunity's Template Division is so effective: it has troops that are around for a while to manage all the antibody templates that have been created – so they are ready for immediate antibody production and memory lymphocyte deployment should the same enemy attack again in the future.

We notice that much of the repair is taking place in an area of murky fluid. The Guide tells us that this is a result of leakage from the inflamed, dilated vessels of Blood and from the many ruptured and dying cells. Initially, because of the enemy's massive invasion, Blood's vessels dilated, stretching their walls and making them quite thin and permeable. This enabled phagocytic and repair troops to pass through those walls to transport necessary nutrients and proteins for healing and repair and to deliver enzymatic chemicals for breaking down foreign material. Now that the initial benefits of dilation and easy transport are no longer of primary significance, the original fluid is contaminated by the leakage of materials from ruptured cells. It appears that this murky fluid may be more of a hazard than a benefit.

The increased flow of Blood has increased the temperature of the area, which in turn increases the speed of some of the chemical reactions and speeds up movement and activity of the phagocytes' cleanup and repair troops.

When I take my eyes off the activity, I see something that I did not want to see – the carnage. It was much easier to watch the cleaning and patching crews than to look at dead bodies and body parts. For emotional comfort, I ask a colleague to explore with me.

We see that a majority of the nerve troops appear to be dead – their bodies ruptured and their extremities ragged. Some are in the process of being engulfed and digested by Macrophages. Of the injured nerve troops that are still alive, a few look as if they could be saved and rehabilitated, others as if they might survive but will never be able to put in a full day's work, and others as if they will surely be dead shortly.

There is a group of nerve troops that appear normal – no evidence of trauma, but absolutely no sign of life. We move closer to look for wounds we might have missed, but find none. They appear to be asleep or stunned. We elect to call the Guide to ask his opinion. He, in turn, calls in two kind of funny-looking fellows from Glia's workforce who are working in the area. The Guide apparently knows them.

They introduce themselves as Oligodendrocytes, part of the Glia, and explain that their primary job is to support and maintain the structure and infrastructure for the CNS, but that they are also responsible for the nerves' nourishment. They are very pleasant to meet and very willing to explain what they are there to do. They even demonstrate how their bodies are designed to transfer materials, nutrients and chemicals directly from Blood's supply conduits to a troop.

We show them some of the nerve troops that we were concerned about – the ones that seem stunned but otherwise rather normal – and ask for their opinion. They immediately bring our attention back to the murky fluid that we had been concerned about earlier, and say, "There is your problem."

The Oligodendrocytes confirm what the Guide described earlier: that although the fluid had initially contained beneficial chemicals needed for the war effort, over the course of the conflict, its composition was significantly altered by elements from ruptured and dying nerve and enemy troops and blood conduits. The fluid now is full of sodium, calcium and potassium in quantities that "shorted out" the electrical circuitry of the nerves' energy supply system. They emphasize the importance of having the vital chemicals in perfect or near-perfect balance, stating that, once the balance is upset, it results in dysfunction or death.

The Oligodendrocytes feel quite sure, however, that, with the cleanup and patch-up programs underway by the highly capable Glia troops, most of the stunned troops will recover fully. They inform us that, even though the Glia troops work for the CNS, they use a chemical communication system, rather than the CNS's electrical communication system. As Oligodendrocytes, they assure us that they are experts in chemistry and the problems associated with imbalance in that area.

At this point, the Guide takes a quick glance at his watch. Time is running short, and he feels it important that we at least take a brief look at the areas in Brain where fighting has been reported, rather than going back through the GI front. He thanks the two Oligodendrocytes for the informative discussion. They ask us to say hello should we meet up with anyone from the Astrocyte Division of Glia. The more talkative of the two explains that Astrocytes do about the same type of work as Oligodendrocytes, except that, because they work in the Brain, they get better pay ("And more time off," quips the quieter one – and then they shake with laughter).

As they leave, the Guide calls us over to chide us for overlooking an important detail of the war related to recovery. With this, he takes us back to look more carefully at the carnage. As we mill around to closer investigate, we come upon an area of stacks of old empty nerve sheaths. The nerves that had lived there had been killed by the enemy and their bodies removed. The sheaths are all that remain. This area is relatively neat, compared to the areas we saw earlier where there was disarray and distortion caused by Inflammation's scarring. The few nerve sheaths that we saw there had been scarred shut.

We ask the Guide what the difference is between the two areas, and he explains that, where the nerves have suffered death by necrosis, we will see disarray and distortion. We are now investigating stacks of nerve sheaths where the nerves have been killed by apoptosis. He also tells us that we are still missing something important.

We search for the clues the Guide told us we missed. At first, we see nothing; then one of us squeals as we see, peeking from the space between two empty nerve sheaths, a wormlike creature, with no visible eyes but a soft cone-like tip, moving rhythmically back and forth. As we watch, the creature finally finds an opening into a nerve sheath and, after a few more searching probes, descends into the tube.

The Guide has a little smile on his face as he listens to our excited chatter. "I hope you can come up with some better scientific terminology when you write up your final report," he teases. "I don't think the committee will be impressed with 'adorable' and 'wiggly thing.'"

By this time, we can see several of these adorable wiggly things. The Guide steps forward to one of them and holds it in his hand, moving aside the stacks of empty sheaths and other material so that we could see how long it is and where it originates. To our surprise, it sprouts from between two plaques of myelin that are insulating a live nerve and not been killed by the virus. As we follow the length of the nerve, we find dozens of similar "axon sprouts" (as the Guide informs us the wiggly things are called) originating along the way. We try to get the axons' attention, but they ignore us. They continue to probe and search at an almost frantic pace.

The Guide is overcome with enthusiasm. Soon he is pointing out one thing and then another, trying to explain to us what is going on. He shows us that the tip of the axon has no eyes: it is a nose cone that specializes in searching for endoneural sheaths that will lead new axon sprouts to orphaned muscle fibers.

He shows us the translucent, soft surface of the nose, through which we can see neatly stacked micro-tubules, positively charged on one end and negatively charged on the other. He tells us that, when they are released, they extend forward and produce a long micro-tubule that will carry the nerve fiber itself. The electrical charges help to move the tubules, position them, and hold them in place.

At this time, a couple of Schwann cells come by and hop onto the sheath that the axon cone had just poked his way into. The Schwanns mark off distances and then start laying out myelin insulation material. As we watch, more and more Schwann cells join them. Each measures off a bit of turf and wraps it with insulation. As they do so, the blood capillaries seem to become more prominent as well.

The Guide approaches the first Schwanns on the scene and asks if they might answer a few questions for us. They warn us that they are very busy and emphasize the supreme importance of their job. And though we have no argument there, it is the way they talk and insist on using the family name that tells us they are a little full of themselves. But they are also full of good information and, ultimately, willing to share it.

They inform us that, as Schwanns, they are part of the Glia and have two primary functions: to produce and wrap myelin insulation around the nerve sheath, as we had observed, and to produce growth hormones to help stimulate the nerve's growth along its way. The more insulation they can apply, the faster and more safely the nerve impulse can travel. We ask them what they did during the battle, before the axons had begun to sprout. One of the Schwanns replies, "Well, I worked with the Cleanup Division as a Phagocyte. That's part of a Glia's responsibility, and I'm a team player."

At this point, we see several Glial cells peeking through holes in the sheath, and the Guide asks to talk to them. They are surprised at his interest but more than willing to tell it as they saw it. Because they live right in the wall of the sheath, they are "where the action is." Like the Schwann cells, these Glia also make growth-stimulation products. They tell us about the overwhelming distances the axons have to grow and how, as Glias, it is their job to provide food, oxygen, and energy to the nerves throughout that entire distance.

One of our teammates asks about transport systems. This creates a frenzy, with all of the Glia trying to talk at once. They inform us that all the proteins, building materials, and the like, are built in the area of the nucleus of the nerve and have to be transported by one of two active transfer systems – a fast system and a slow system. They indicate that it would take years for things to get back and forth between the nucleus of the nerve and the footpad on the muscle fiber if it were not for these very simple and mechanical active transport systems.

Then someone asks whether it is true that the polio virus is actually carried by the axon's own transport system up to the nucleus where it infects and kills the nerve. The question catches the Glia off guard. Finally, one steps forward. His answer is forthright, but tinged with a bit of embarrassment and apology.

"Yes, it is true. But as things are, I don't think it could have been prevented. You see, the virus is very small. It is about the same size as the proteins and building materials we carry back and forth on the transport system all the time. So, once the virus finds the PVR and gets into the nerve, all it has to do is climb on the transport, which will carry it directly to the nucleus. I'm sorry, but I can only think of one thing that might prevent that, and that is vaccination. Then the Immunity Division's antibodies would have bonded with the virus and prevented it from climbing aboard. We have spent a lot of time thinking about this, but other than getting Immunity involved early, there is no way to prevent it."

We all share a reflective moment.

Anxious to change the subject, one Glia, impressed by our fancy magnification glasses, suggests that we take a quick peek into one of the sheaths that was being restored. Looking down that tube, we can see that the micro-tubules that had been stored in the nose cone were already being laid out and that there were more, along with other building materials, coming down the slow-transit system. In some of the sheaths, neurofilaments are already in place. We also see capillaries carrying blood and oxygen. There were some Oligodendrocytes supporting the vessels and neurofilaments by transferring nutrients from the blood vessels to the nerve fibers. What they are accomplishing is amazing.

The Guide checks the time and informs us that we need to start back soon. Several of the Glia express dismay that we will not get to see the axon actually reach and attach to the orphaned muscle fiber, so they brief us on what will happen.

They explain that a blister of Nerve Cell Adhesion Molecule (N-CAM) was already sitting on the surface of the muscle fiber, beckoning and directing the axon toward it. Once the axon establishes contact with the N-CAM blister, the attachment for the footpad of the axon will develop, and the muscle fiber should be able to function again.

They then lean forward and whisper, as if sharing a secret, that there really is no physical connection between the axon's footpad and the muscle fiber, but rather just a space. They confide that vesicles manufactured in the nucleus are filled with a chemical called *acetylcholine* that drips from the vesicle onto the receptor site on the muscle fiber, and that that is how the muscle gets its direction, or stimulation. (The Guide tells us later that this point has been argued scientifically for years. Seeing it firsthand would have given us bragging rights.)

Although we haven't been able to complete his entire agenda, the Guide seems satisfied with what we have been able to see. He finds a passage into the Cerebral Spinal Canal, and we start our swim upward. It is warm and pleasant, but requires a bit more effort on our part than the previous trip in one of Blood's vessels. We find the opening in the BBB without difficulty and help each other out. We step onto Tonsils as we leave and march single file toward the Oral entrance along a narrow pathway called the Buccal Fold. We soon find a rhythm, and the thrill of the day's events make us feel like warriors returning from victory. We must be a hilarious site as we emerge from the Body's mouth and march the few steps to the Miniaturizing Chamber, which had been reverse-programmed (and hopefully sanitized) since its morning use next to Anal Pass.

What is even more hilarious is the six minutes it takes to get de-miniaturized, which starts with a surprising bunch of snaps, pops, and rips as buttons, seams, and Velcro give way. We all are giggling as we emerge full-sized from the chamber. There are hugs, handshakes, and promises to get together again shortly. Whether we will or not, only time will tell, but we all know that today was a once-in-a-lifetime experience.

Part Two

CHAPTER 8

POST POLIO: AN INTRODUCTION

Post Polio is not a continuation of the polio infection. It has nothing to do with any ongoing or recurrent activity of the original polio virus. In 1949, polio went through me like a Kansas tornado. It hit fast and hard – decisively and destructively – and then was gone. Those of us who were able to breathe, swallow, and maintain adequate blood pressure and heart rhythm during that brief but critical period survived. Recovery began the moment the virus was eliminated, and everything that followed was, by definition, *post* the polio infection.

I had put up with polio's initial attack, suffered the consequences, and accepted the limitations it left me. So when decades later I began to suffer from unusual muscle fatigue and weakness – and later, pain, tiredness, and other frustrating symptoms – I felt blindsided. I thought I'd held up my end of the deal. And now there was more to come?

I was not alone in thinking I was "done" with polio. With the remarkable results of the immunization campaign of the 1950s, much of the medical community had believed that polio was behind us as a nation. But when in the late 1970s large numbers of polio survivors began reporting similar complaints of pain, weakness, and tiredness – decades after recovering from the acute infection – a small number of researchers took note. Thanks to their persistence and diligence, much has been learned about the late effects of polio, or what I will refer to here as the Post-Polio Stage.

Manifestations of Post Polio

Given what you've learned in earlier chapters about the physiology of polio infection and recovery, you will not be too surprised at some of the symptoms most frequently experienced by polio persons as they age: weakness, pain, tiredness, and sometimes difficulty breathing and swallowing. The inherent limitations of recovery from paralytic polio foreshadowed the challenges we are most likely to face as the natural attrition of age takes its toll. When these symptoms became significant enough that they were affecting our daily living, we had entered the Post-Polio Stage.

In the ensuing chapters, I will address these manifestations of Post Polio in greater depth. First, we will look closely at what I think of as the trio of primary manifestations: muscle fatigue and weakness, pain, and tiredness. We will also take a look at difficulty breathing and swallowing – another frequent issue for aging survivors of polio. After a review of these symptoms, we'll dig into some collateral concerns and other aspects of incorporating post-polio considerations into our daily lives.

While each may experience Post Polio differently, an awareness of these late effects is important for effectively managing our healthcare and quality of life as we age. Recognizing that your history of polio may be playing a role in your current medical condition, and being able to articulate that to your physicians, family, and caregivers are critical pieces of your self-advocacy.

Post-Polio Syndrome

In 1984, researchers organized an international conference on the late effects of polio at the Warm Springs Rehabilitation Center in Georgia. Experts met to investigate the reported symptoms that were appearing in those who had survived the polio epidemic many years prior. It was at this conference that the term *post-polio syndrome* was coined. Subsequent conferences and research have served to refine the definition of the syndrome.

Post-polio syndrome is considered a new condition that affects survivors of polio decades after their initial infection. The criteria for diagnosis of post-polio syndrome include:

- Prior paralytic poliomyelitis with evidence of motor neuron loss, as confirmed by history of the acute paralytic illness, signs of residual weakness and atrophy of muscles on neuromuscular examination, and signs of nerve damage on electromyography (EMG). Rarely, persons have subclinical paralytic polio, described as a loss of motor neurons during acute polio but with no obvious deficit. That prior polio now needs to be confirmed with an EMG. Also, a reported history of non-paralytic polio may

be inaccurate.
- A period of partial or complete functional recovery after acute paralytic poliomyelitis, followed by an interval (usually 15 years or more) of stable neuromuscular function.
- Gradual onset of progressive and persistent new muscle weakness or abnormal muscle fatigability (decreased endurance), with or without generalized fatigue, muscle atrophy, or muscle and joint pain. Onset may at times follow trauma, surgery, or a period of inactivity, and can appear to be sudden. Less commonly, symptoms attributed to PPS include new problems with breathing or swallowing.
- Symptoms that persist for at least a year.
- Exclusion of other neuromuscular, medical, and orthopedic problems as causes of symptoms.

Modified from: *Post-Polio Syndrome: Identifying Best Practices in Diagnosis & Care.* March of Dimes, 2001.[23]

A post-polio syndrome diagnosis is a diagnosis of exclusion. In other words, it requires that no other conditions are causing or contributing to the symptoms. This means that fewer people will be diagnosed with post-polio syndrome than will be impacted by the late effects of polio. Regardless of whether you are technically within the criteria for post-polio

---

[23] Office of Communications and Public Liaison, National Institute of Neurological Disorders and Stroke, National Institutes of Health, "Post-Polio Syndrome Fact Sheet," *NIH Publication No. 06-4030,* last updated June 6, 2011 (Bethesda: National Institute of Neurological Disorders and Stroke, 2011).

syndrome, the late effects of polio (also known as post-polio sequelae) may be affecting your health and should be a factor in your health management.[24]

---

[24] Within the post-polio literature, there are inconsistencies in the use of the terms "syndrome," "sequelae," and "late effects of polio." I have tried to maintain consistency in this book, using "post-polio syndrome" to refer specifically to the condition defined by the criteria set out above, and speaking more generally of "Post Polio" or the "Post-Polio Stage" to refer to the period during which one experiences the late effects of polio (or post-polio sequelae), regardless of whether they meet the criteria for post-polio syndrome.

CHAPTER 9

WEAKNESS

Weakness was a by-product of the polio infection. It affected all survivors to some degree. For some, it was so minimal, initially, that it was clinically imperceptible. For others, we've lived with making accommodations for our weakness ever since. Since the last virus particle met its demise, I've had to push myself up from sitting, take the stairs one at a time, and get the kids to pick the newspaper up from off the doorstep. It was only much later that these accommodations became obviously insufficient. More was needed. I added bracing, crutches, handrails, and other modifications to my environment. Weakness had become something I could feel and others could see. At this point, I had to accept that I was in the Post-Polio Stage.

Post-polio weakness is a muscular thing; it is the direct result of *muscle fatigue*. For those of us with Post Polio, muscle fatigue relates to our muscles' limited ability to perform work. Accepting that as the definition will make our understanding and treatment of post-polio weakness much easier.[25]

---

[25] Although muscle fatigue does not need to be present to make the diagnosis of post-polio syndrome, when it is present, it can be the most disabling part of the syndrome.

Peripheral vs. Central Muscular Fatigue

Muscle fatigue can be broken down into two types: *peripheral* and *central*. It may be helpful to look at two different definitions of "fatigue" from the *Merriam-Webster Dictionary*: (1) "weariness or exhaustion from labor, exertion, or stress," and (2) "the temporary loss of power to respond that is induced in a sensory receptor or motor end organ by continued stimulation."[26]

The first definition is more helpful in understanding *peripheral fatigue*. Peripheral fatigue originates in the skeletal muscle and involves only the muscle and its chemistry. It results from labor, exertion, or stress; it is physiologically and chemically manifested within the muscle and clinically recognized by us as weakness. Many of us with Post Polio experience peripheral fatigue with more frequency and after less exertion as our functional neuromuscular mass is reduced.

In contrast, *central fatigue* is caused by the muscle's inability to maintain strength throughout repeated contractions – not because the muscle is running low on fuel but because the impulse that is being sent to it by the brain is weakening. Central fatigue is therefore more consistent with the dictionary's second definition of fatigue.

Muscle Fiber Types

To better understand how our post-polio muscles work, we need some familiarity with skeletal muscle fibers, their

---

[26] *Merriam-Webster Online Dictionary, s.v. "fatigue,"* 2011, accessed February 15, 2011, http://www.merriam-webster.com.

fueling systems, and how they are affected by our polio.[27]

We will focus on the two primary skeletal muscle fiber types: Type I and Type IIb.[28] There are a multitude of other names for these two fiber types, used to describe the metabolic and/or functional variations. I guess which terminology you use may relate to your age, where you trained, or whether you are a muscle physiologist, a metabolic chemist, or work the counter at KFC.

Type I muscle fiber	=	slow oxidation	=	slow twitch	=	fatigue-resistant	=	dark meat
Type IIb muscle fiber	=	fast glycolytic	=	fast twitch	=	easily fatigued	=	white meat

Type I muscle fiber is extremely dense and contains a variety of elements: lots of *myoglobin*, which carries oxygen into the muscle cells, as well as *myosin* and *actin*, the contracting protein elements of the muscle cell. Dark meat also has many *mitochondria*, which facilitate the production of *adenosine triphosphate (ATP)*, an energy-rich molecule that stores the power we need for function. These elements are surrounded by dense networks of tiny blood vessels (capillaries)

---

[27] We are referring only to *skeletal muscle* here. Skeletal muscle is also sometimes called *motor-type muscle* or *striated muscle*. Other types of muscles are *cardiac muscle* (which causes the heart to pump) and *smooth muscle* (found in the intestine, bladder, blood vessels, eyeball, and skin).

[28] There is a spectrum of other fiber types, but for our purposes we will focus on Type I and Type IIb.

that bring oxygen and nutrients to the cell and carry its metabolic wastes away. All of these increase the cell's density and darken its appearance.

We can think of Type I muscle fiber as heavily industrialized; it has all the machinery necessary for the manufacture of its own fuel. With the help of oxygen, imported glycogen and fat are converted to ATP, making Type I muscle fibers fatigue-resistant and available for the long haul. This is what makes it the desired muscle fiber of the endurance athlete. Like the Energizer Bunny, if properly paced, Type I muscle fibers can go on and on and on.

Type IIb muscle fibers have their fuel in the form of glycogen stored within the cells as well as the chemicals (*glycolytic enzymes*) necessary to break the glycogen down into ATP fuel. These muscle fibers do not need the industrial quantities of capillaries or large numbers of mitochondria that darken the Type I muscle. Type IIb fibers' fuel sources, although very limited, are already within their cell walls and are available for an immediate response. Because the quantity of their fuel supply is small, however, they can function at maximum capacity for only a short period of time. To their advantage, these cells contain more *myofibrils* (little contracting muscle fibrils) and higher activity from *ATPase enzymes* (enzymes that release energy by breaking down ATP). This enables them to generate much greater force quickly. Greater force and greater speed are what differentiate the Type IIb muscle fiber from the Type I.

We humans do not have white meat and dark meat as does the chicken. Our muscles are a mixture of the different types of fibers, so neither color predominates. However, as you might expect, we are likely to find more of the white meat, fast-twitch, Type IIb fibers in, for example, the muscles of our upper extremities and eyelids, to accommodate their quick decisive functions. And we would find more of the dark meat, slow-twitch, Type I fibers in the muscles of the back and lower extremities whose lifting, holding, and stabilizing functions have greater need for endurance and resistance to fatigue.

Muscle Fuel

Muscle fatigue is a normal phenomenon. It is a natural, protective mechanism that tells you that muscle fuel is starting to run out and an alternate strategy might need to be considered. You either have to stop the activity or find another source of fuel. In this way, *acute* (sudden onset) fatigue is much like acute pain; it tells you that something has to be done – now! Acute muscle weakness and the resulting fatigue may go so far as to make you fall or otherwise step out of the race, rather than allowing us to be placed at greater risk. So, unless you are racing to escape a tiger or other threat to your life, fatigue is probably working on your behalf – protecting you from overexertion and the potential hazards that could result.

Availability

The development of muscle fatigue relates most directly to the availability of muscle fuel and how it is used. Muscle cells have variable amounts of ATP fuel precursors stored and available for immediate use. A normal human muscle (a mixture of both Type I and Type IIb muscle fibers) has enough stored ATP fuel to power maximal muscle contractions for about two or three seconds. After that, a second source of ATP fuel produced from *phosphocreatine* – also stored within its cells – will power the muscle for another twenty to thirty seconds. Then, if available, *intra-cellular glycogen* can be used to extend the muscle's power for possibly another two to three minutes.

Note that, up to this point, the fueling of the muscle has not required the use of oxygen and has used only the immediately available, intracellular sources of ATP fuel. We can therefore safely assume that the Type IIb muscle fibers were carrying the bulk of the load. Though the maximal performance time for this muscle is very brief, the power is immediately available to serve our fight-or-flight instincts, enabling us to strike quickly and get out of there fast, to run for a tree or cave to hide in, or to duck or blink the eyes to prevent injury. We don't have much time, but that immediate availability is very basic to our survival.

To function beyond this, muscles need to have oxygen. It is during this phase that the expertise of the heavily industrialized, Type I muscle fibers comes into play. By adding oxygen, imported *glycogen* will produce enough ATP fuel to keep the muscle contracting at near maximum rate for another thirty to sixty minutes. When these glycogen stores are exhausted, with oxygen still available, imported *fat* can produce ATP fuel and keep the muscle contracting while the fat supply holds out.

It's kind of like the five speeds in an automatic transmission; although the power and speed of the vehicle are related to switching from one gear to another (instead of from one fuel source to another), the transition is similarly smooth and efficient and is dependent on the load and stress as related to time. As you can see, there are different fuel supplies for different types and durations of effort, and the chemical pathways to muscle fatigue may vary because of this.

Toxicity

So far, I've focused on the role of *fuel availability* in muscle function and fatigue. However, when we produce and burn fuel, we create *waste products* and those waste products, too, can affect muscle performance.

One way that waste products are created is through repetitive muscle activity. In a 100-meter sprint, the runner will reach maximum speed at about sixty meters; after that, the speed begins to decline. In a 1997 article, muscle physiologists D. G. Allen, J. Lännergren, and H. Westerblad posited that this decline may occur because of the accumulation of phosphate that results when phosphocreatine is used as a source for ATP fuel.[29] The toxic effect of this phosphate by-product reduces the muscles' ability to produce force and is a cause of muscle fatigue.

Just as there is more than one way to skin the proverbial cat, there is also more than one way to poison a muscle.

---

[29] D G Allen, J Lännergren, and H Westerblad, "The role of ATP in the regulation of intracellular Ca2+ release in single fibres of mouse skeletal muscle," *The Journal of Physiology* 498.3 (1997): 587-600.

When a muscle is contracted, it squeezes the blood vessels within, preventing free blood flow, depriving the muscle of adequate oxygen and nutrients, and causing metabolic wastes to accumulate. Skeletal muscle is not designed for sustained contraction; it requires intermittent relaxation to refresh the nutrient supply and flush out the waste products. (A charley horse is an example of a muscle's response to sustained contraction; until muscle relaxation occurs and freer blood flow is restored, that muscle can be a real pain.) With sustained contraction, waste products accumulate, leading to muscle fatigue.

Weight lifting is an extreme example of sustained muscle contraction. For the weight lifter, fatigue may set in, in a matter of seconds. In addition to the rapid exhaustion of oxygen-independent fuels (glycogen, ATP, and phosphocreatine), the intense muscle contraction squeezes off the supply of oxygen and nutrients to the cells and interferes with the removal of the metabolic by-product, namely, *potassium*. The elevated level of potassium interferes with the penetration of action potentials (nerve impulses) into the deeper muscle fiber parts, causing reduced calcium levels. Decreased calcium leads to a decrease in contractile force of the deeper fibers of the muscle, which we recognize as fatigue.

The Making of an Impulse

If ever anything were created by committee, it would have to be the impulse the muscle receives from the brain. This impulse is the result of data coming from myriad sensory organs throughout the mind and body. Data on every conceivable subject – temperature, position, chemical levels, mood, and the like – are delivered to the brain for processing. The mental and physical demands and capacities of the moment will therefore affect the location, type, and intensity of that impulse. For example, the brain may send a heightened impulse to facilitate escape or it may suggest a slowdown in activity for the well-being of the muscle or the body general. We have to assume that the final command the brain gives to the muscle is in the momentary best interest of the body.

One would expect, with all the input that goes into the development of an impulse, that, once an impulse has been determined, it will be final. For the most part, that is true, but the impulse can face many challenges on its journey from inception to destination – and some of these may influence the content of the impulse itself.

Think of a nerve impulse originating in the motor area at the top of the brain. First, it must travel through the brain and spinal cord where thirty trillion or so synapses, or switchings, occur every second, posing a possible threat to that new impulse. If it successfully makes it through the brain and spinal cord, the impulse is handed over to the motor nerve designed to carry its message to the designated muscle fiber.

The distance the impulse must travel via the motor nerve, from spinal cord to muscle, is relatively long, and along the way it may be exposed to a multitude of adverse influences from outside the nervous system: low oxygen levels as might be found in severe emphysema, chemical imbalances associated with advanced kidney disease, temperature changes, toxins, and physical trauma, to name only a few. You can begin to see how many ways that impulse could be modified during the course of its travel from its origin in the brain to its destination at the terminal footpad of the axon sprout, where it is to communicate with the muscle.

Perhaps we can now better understand why central fatigue may be more pronounced in those of us with Post Polio. Central fatigue is not due to muscular dysfunction, but rather is related to the progressively weakening impulses sent to the muscle by the brain. The reason for the weakening impulses is that the impulse a muscle receives *from* the brain is a response to information that sensors in the muscle have sent *to* the brain. So, when the motor cortex receives a message from a muscle that has been compromised, such as in a post-polio person, the brain may try to protect the compromised muscle by electing not to drive the motor neurons with a steady level of vigor. Instead, it delivers a progressively weakening controlling impulse to that muscle, limiting the person's ability to sustain activity.

Treatment and Prevention

Muscles start to fatigue at the onset of activity; it's not something that only happens after a certain amount or type of activity or after a defined period of time has passed. The treatment of muscle fatigue is rest. There are two types of recovery from muscle fatigue: fast and slow. Both require rest.

The faster type of recovery requires only a few minutes and is related to the time it takes to replenish phosphocreatine and glycogen stores in the cell and to wash out accumulated lactic acid and other wastes. In my case, this fast component seems to relate to the times I felt fatigued after being physically active. I would lie down to rest and then, after only a few minutes, would ask myself, "What am I lying down for? I don't feel tired anymore."

The slower type of recovery follows excessive use, after which the muscles may feel heavy, a bit painful, and weakened, requiring a few days of rest. The muscles will perform, but it seems to require mental effort and coaxing; it is almost as if they have to be told to take each step. This is thought to be from defects in calcium release.[30]

During my years of practice, I was able to work hard in my office all day without fatiguing because my exam rooms were compact and conveniently equipped. Except for an occasional seventy-foot jaunt to lab or x-ray, I rarely walked more than twenty feet at a time and would go all day without noticing muscle fatigue. My muscles apparently had plenty of recovery time between those short runs. However, as I approached my fortieth year post-polio, I began to dread making rounds at the nursing homes and hospitals. The hallways in these facilities were 100–300 feet long, the patient beds were low and difficult to bend over, and there was no resting between patients. On those occasions, I did notice muscle fatigue; however, I was usually in a situation where I could modify my activity. If I could share the load with my nurse practitioner, or split the nursing-home rounds over two

---

[30] Andrew M. Bellinger, Steven Reiken, Miroslav Dura, et al. "Remodeling of ryanodine receptor complex causes 'leaky' channels: a molecular mechanism for decreased exercise capacity," *Proceedings of the National Academy of Sciences of the United States of America* vol. 105 no. 6 (2008): 2198–2202, doi:10.1073/pnas.0711074105.

days, or sit down while reviewing a chart or taking a patient's history, I could limit the stress, avoid exhaustion, and recover promptly. Usually, by the time I got back to my office, I was good for the rest of the day. This experience seems to relate to the fast component of recovery.

It wasn't until after my back surgery that I had significant experience with the slower type of recovery. Up to that point, my polio weakness had never allowed me to exert myself to the point of protein damage. My reduced neuromuscular mass worked in my favor, fatiguing me before I could do too much damage to the little muscle I had left. However, following surgery, just trying to regain my pre-surgical level of strength and activity with my reduced muscle mass proved to be so overwhelming that my muscles were spent, and it was then that I experienced the "slower" recovery.

Because muscular fatigue, whether central or peripheral, will by definition be relieved with rest, rest might be used as a simple diagnostic test. A relatively prompt response to rest, often just lying down or sitting down to get the weight off the muscles, will differentiate fatigued muscles from depression, sleep deprivation, mental exhaustion, or tiredness associated with acute or chronic illness.

Another way to differentiate muscular fatigue from, let's say, tiredness or depression, is to consider the systems involved. Our muscles are designed to work twenty-four hours a day with only brief periods of rest for eliminating waste and refueling. The brain, on the other hand, needs prolonged periods of rest, six to eight hours out of every twenty-four. Exhaustion of the brain, as might be found in mental stress, depression, and chemical imbalances associated with other diseases, is manifested by the sensation of tiredness; it may take days or weeks to resolve and will require the correction of the underlying problem – not just rest.

Quite often, in the literature on Post Polio, the symptoms are not differentiated from symptoms associated with aging, such as weakness, tiredness, depression, cardiopulmonary dysfunction, or joint pain. As a consequence, statements that are made to look like "polio fact" actually apply equally to our aging, non-polio peers. The disability of weakness for those of us with Post Polio is related to the ease of fatigue production as a direct result of the markedly reduced amount of functional neuromuscular mass that we have available to do the things we need to and want to do.

The body is not going to make major changes in its basic fueling and metabolic recovery systems just for us, but the limitations of these fueling and metabolic recovery systems may be severely tested by post-polio muscles whose nerve supply is lacking reserves, whose recovery fibers are severely overworked, whose axon sprouts may not be perfect replicas of the original nerve either anatomically or metabolically, and whose workload may be further increased because the team's players have been changed.[31] Just performing the necessary activities of daily living may pose as much of a physical challenge for the post-polio person as a rigorous training routine does for a competitive athlete. Our post-polio muscle fatigue and the resulting weakness are directly related to having to do, or trying to do, too much with too little.

---

[31] Please refer to "The Reinnervation Phase" in chapter 5.

Chapter 10

Pain

As I began writing this chapter, I had been having pain for the past several days and decided it was probably a good time to write on the topic. Most of the time, I can feel, in almost all of my body, not really pain, but more of an *awareness*. At this moment, however, I am having real pain … in my wrists, thumbs, elbows, knees, shoulders, upper thighs, and low back. When I first stand up, the pain in the low back is very uncomfortable and remains so until I am upright for several minutes, and then it may all but disappear. Upper back, neck, and right hip pain are also present right now. At times like these, a good question might be: Where *don't* I have pain? Many of us who suffer from post-polio pain have a couple of other questions: Is the pain I now experience part of my polio? Was it caused by my polio? Where does Post Polio come into the picture?

The Polio Component

Some of us are old enough to be familiar with the term "shimmy" as it relates to the wobbling of a loose wheel on a car. Others of us may get a more vivid definition of the term if we remember the song "I Wish I Could Shimmy Like My Sister Kate." Although the recollections of Kate shimmying on the dance floor are more pleasant, the first illustration is probably more appropriate for post-polio joint disease. Usually, when the wheel first begins to shimmy or wobble, the shaky movement is almost indiscernible; however, if not properly addressed, it will further damage the wheel, which eventually may cause it to break down completely.

That is what happened to me. At my point of maximum recovery, my polio infection had left me enough muscle and tendon to support my joints – but only just enough. And although I was able to function adequately at that time, there was already too little support surrounding those joints to provide the stability I needed for the loads that I placed on them. Though the joints outwardly appeared stable, they were already a little loose. There was simply not enough neuromuscular mass to keep the joints stabilized. With time, the damage to the joint became more apparent, often with deformity, disability, and, eventually, pain.

Pain Comes in Two Flavors

Acute Pain

Acute pain is a friend. It's always there to warn us and protect us from harm, be it a hot stove or a sharp knife. The nerve ending sensing the threat will first send a message to the motor nerves that initiates withdrawal from the noxious stimulus, and at almost the same time, the brain and spinal cord will get the same report. Therefore, in addition to instituting the withdrawal response, there follows the interpretation by the brain and spinal cord that the noxious stimulus is probably something we should put on record to make sure we avoid it in the future. For example, if you have been burned on a stove and later come across a stove, you will either avoid it or approach it differently, because you have learned to respect the stove as a source of injury.

Once the body has sustained an injury and withdrawn from the source of that injury, pain takes on a role of a different nature, a protective role. Now the pain we feel is produced by the injury itself and is coming from within the body, so there is no longer a need for a withdrawal response. Instead, the brain now recognizes a need to heal, so it initiates behaviors that favor the healing process. Such behaviors may include limiting activity, seeking warmth and shelter, and physically protecting and supporting the injured area. For many animals, licking the wound would be included in a list of healing and protective behaviors. We do it too. There isn't one of us who hasn't licked or kissed a cut, abrasion, or contusion of a finger or thumb. It is often the first thing we do, suggesting that it is an innate, reflex behavior for us as well. As parents, we often kiss our children's "owies" to make them feel better, and interestingly, it usually works.

As described above, when healthy tissue is disturbed, acute pain develops in that location to tell us that something is wrong and needs to be corrected. The acute pain will stop as soon as the inflammation related to the injury has been controlled. It may be a matter of seconds or minutes, as in the case of an acute muscle strain or a poke in the eye, or it may persist to some degree for weeks, as in the case of an infected knee joint or a bruised tailbone.

Neuropathic Pain

There is another type of pain – neuropathic pain – that is malicious. Neuropathic pain is not our friend. It is chronic, lasting, by definition, six months to a lifetime. It may follow an injury or infection, but in a large percentage of cases, a history of such cannot be obtained. Chronic pain of this type may be located far away from the site of an injury or infection, and it may even have a pattern that defies its origin on an anatomical basis. In other words, you may not be able to trace along the nerve anatomy and connect the location of the chronic pain to the source; it may even be bilateral which is very hard to explain on an anatomical basis.

Neuropathic pain can come in many forms. It may be in the form of an exaggerated response, for example, severe pain resulting from what should have been recognized as a light touch. I had a patient who could not shave the right side of his face because of the severe pain produced by just touching it. Another patient, an elderly lady with scalp pain following shingles, could not comb her hair because of the pain produced. Phantom limb syndrome, which very occasionally follows the amputation of an extremity, refers to the sensation of the extremity still being present after amputation. The sensation is usually that of pain, though it may be felt as tingling, a numb sensation, burning, or some other distortion of what we think of as pain.[32]

---

[32] There are four ways that a sensory nerve may respond to injury or inflammation. *Anesthesia*, or numbness, refers to the absence of sensation after injury. *Paresthesias* are abnormal sensations, such as tingling or burning, that occur in the absence of any obvious stimulation. *Dysesthesia* refers to an unexpected or abnormal sensation that occurs following the stimulation of a

Neuropathic pain may occur at the extremes of intensity, from almost-indiscernible tingling to excruciating, debilitating pain. Probably the nicest thing that can be said about chronic neuropathic pain is that its lack of response to opiates and nonsteroidal anti-inflammatory drugs has led to the current wave of research that is giving us a new understanding of pain, its basis, and how we approach and treat it.

Holding Still

With reference to my pain of recent years, its severity is variable, and episodes of it come and go. When I'm having an episode, I move slowly, my glass is half empty, and I'm not much fun to have around. Though my pain is often precipitated by periods of excessive or unusual activity, for me, it is just as likely, or even more likely, that pain will result from inactivity or, more accurately, *non-movement* – times when I am required to *hold still*.

Holding still requires the use of your muscles to stabilize and maintain a position, and that can take a tremendous amount of energy. If I am sitting at the computer or doing anything else that keeps my head and neck in one position for a prolonged period of time, I will notice neck and shoulder pain. For me, pain will also follow periods of prolonged sitting, especially if the chair support is not good. Prolonged standing without movement will also trigger a painful episode. In

---

nerve or group of nerves. A fourth type of abnormal response is a greater amount of pain or discomfort than would normally be expected when a particular nerve is stimulated; this is called *allodynia*.

retrospect, the severe leg and back pain I started having while standing on a riser and singing in the church choir was one of the first things to suggest to me that I might have what had just recently been reported and named post-polio syndrome.

Often, partial or complete relief from pain caused by maintaining position can be achieved almost immediately by changing position. This puts the workload on a different group of muscles and tendons. Remember that skeletal muscle is designed to contract, then relax. It is not designed for sustained contraction. Normally, when one is forced to be in one position for a prolonged period of time, he or she automatically and imperceptibly adjusts to shift the workload back and forth from one neuromuscular unit to another. This gives the working unit a chance to rest, refuel, and rid itself of metabolic waste before it is its turn to contract again. For those with Post Polio, however, there are not enough neuromuscular units in reserve to allow for this constant shifting of the workload. Without the reserves, our neuromuscular units are given no reprieve and have no choice but to remain in sustained contraction. As with a charley horse, the longer the contraction is sustained, the more painful the event.

Disuse

By early 2007, I had developed a large lumbar disc herniation that produced a classic pattern of pain and numbness in my back and leg. The disc was surgically removed, and its pain and numbness disappeared. However, five or six days after the surgery, I began having low back pain of another type. Post-operative weakness and lack of support in my low back led to abnormal tendon and muscle strain of the tissues in that area. I believe this weakness – and the resulting pain – were caused by the period of disuse during my surgery and recovery time. When muscles are not used, levels of actin and myosin (essential contractile proteins) are diminished, and weakness ensues. The amount of muscle stabilizing my back and extremities was so diminished that it took only a short time of disuse to render it too weak to do its job. Exercise strengthens a muscle by increasing its content of actin and myosin.[33] It took three months of exercise before my back was strong enough to control this pain.

Compensation

After this surgery I also began having more pain and discomfort in my arms, shoulders, and neck. Because of the weakness in my back and legs, I needed the use of my hands and arms to lift me in and out of chairs and bed, placing damaging pressure on my shoulder, arm, and neck muscles. My situation also required heavy use of crutches and walkers; this put enormous pressure on the ulnar, median, and radial nerves, permanently damaging those nerves and causing chronic numbness and pain in the fingers and hands – a neuropathic pain that will most likely be with me for the rest of my life.

Much of the post-polio pain I now have relates to

---

[33] As discussed in chapter 14, exercise for those of us with Post Polio should be undertaken in consultation with our healthcare professionals and with our individual polio impacts in mind; for some of us, it may not look like traditional "exercise" at all.

degenerative osteoarthritic changes in my joints; however, it is very likely that the joint disease I am experiencing is not primarily related to my polio history. As a physician, I have seen hundreds of x-rays of low backs, necks, thumbs, wrists, knees, and hips of people my age and younger who have never had polio and whose x-rays look no better, on average, than mine. As a matter of fact, I am quite sure that the level of degenerative joint disease that I have developed over time is quite comparable to that of my non-polio peers. But, certainly, my polio history plays a large part in the amount of pain that I have in those joints.

Polio left me with an inadequate amount of muscle mass to stabilize and protect my diseased joints. That polio weakness, coupled with the weakness relative to my own aging, has resulted in an exorbitant amount of stress placed on the joints and the tendons and muscles surrounding them. Any increase in stress or strain on such joints will produce pain.

More to the Story

Much of post-polio pain can be explained, directly or indirectly, by the diminished neuromuscular mass left by the polio infection and further diminished by the natural attrition of aging. But that doesn't explain why, when I abuse my arthritic back, for example, I not only experience pain in my back but also pain and increased tenderness in joints, tendons, and muscles in areas far away from the site of the initiating pain – areas that, prior to this time, had not been causing discomfort. I may even note pain in my teeth when chewing a cracker, or I may have urinary burning and urgency but no symptoms to suggest an infection. What is going on, and how do we treat it? Those are good questions.

Medical science is expanding our understanding of pain and its treatment. Researchers are finding interrelationships between immunity, inflammation, and our genes as well as our peripheral and central nervous systems that, once fully understood, may explain why we have pain and how it relates to fatigue, weakness, depression, and attrition of age.

Pain can be produced by direct injury to a nerve or by injury to tissues adjacent to that nerve. Inflammation arising at the injury site will activate immune cells to produce pro-inflammatory chemicals called *cytokines*.[34] Cytokines circulating in the immediate area of the injury will stimulate local sensory nerves (pain receptor nerves) and produce pain. When tissue is injured, it becomes "sensitized": its threshold for pain is reduced, and its sensory nerves become more susceptible to cytokines (and, therefore, pain) in the future.

When large amounts of pro-inflammatory cytokines are produced as a result of an injury, infection, or stress, the blood may circulate those cytokines throughout the body where they can react with sensitized tissues and nerve cells that are either in peripheral tissues (such as an arthritic joint) or in the central nervous tissues (brain or spinal cord). So now we see why I may be experiencing pain in the neck, arms, knees and even experiencing nonspecific tiredness and despondency, even though the precipitating event was the injury to my back. The pro-inflammatory cytokines circulated by the

---

[34] The inflammation can also commission various non-immune cells in the injury area to function as immune cells, increasing the number of cells that produce cytokines.

blood augment the immune/inflammatory activity already present in arthritic joints that, before this time, may have been completely or relatively asymptomatic.

Dealing with Post-Polio Pain

When I put too much stress on my body, I can expect my joints, tendons, and muscles to complain. So the first thing I do is find the area of stress and then try to correct the situation that is causing that stress. As I've said, often it is just a matter of changing position. Sitting in one position in a chair with poor support is a major cause of pain for me. Changing positions or activities will often relieve this type of pain in very short order.

If the pain becomes more frequent and arises with less provocation, I begin to suspect that it is related to weakness rather than to position. I may have already been feeling some increased generalized weakness. Usually, if I get back into my exercise program and restore my strength to my maintenance level, it will reduce or eliminate the pain.

For many years, I noted that, if I gained five to seven pounds, I would notice pain in my left knee. When I lost the weight, the discomfort disappeared. So, if pain in my back and legs becomes a problem, I pay attention to my diet for two or three weeks and get rid of any excess weight that I have gained.

Pain and weakness in my lower back and legs is often accompanied or closely followed by pain in my hands, wrists, elbows, and shoulders related to the increased burden placed on them from having to lift my weakened body out of chairs, etc. In this case, I look for a higher chair with padded armrests that I can almost step out of rather than hoisting my 165 pounds up and out of a lower one. If a higher chair is not available, I will use two or three pillows to give the seat some height. To protect my hands, I use a length of soft, foam, water pipe insulation to wrap around the handles of my walker and crutches and then wrap that with black electrical tape. It works very well.

Personally, I am not a very good pill taker, but I do take medication to control episodes of severe pain. I am quite accepting of the fact that I will have some degree of discomfort and do not expect medication to make me totally pain-free. Part of that attitude comes from my understanding of the mechanical causes of post-polio pain. Experience has taught me that changing position, increasing support, and reducing stress, both physical and mental, will usually reduce or eliminate most of my pain.

It isn't appropriate for me to outline a program of medication or other treatment for obvious reasons. I am not your physician, so I do not know the nature of your pain and disability. However, the subject of medications is important, so I will share a few thoughts.

Nonsteroidal anti-inflammatory drugs (NSAIDs) can be of some benefit, but they are not without risks. The advantage of NSAIDs is that they have a painkilling effect in addition to their anti-inflammatory effect. The risk arises from the effect of excess NSAID on the system. Excess dosages can result, for example, when a person takes the full NSAID dosage for pain relief and unwittingly gets a large additional amount of the NSAID in an over-the-counter cold, headache, or arthritis medication.[35] Such excess can lead to kidney or gastrointestinal damage or adverse cardiovascular effects. Moreover, it may take two or three weeks to get the full anti-inflammatory effect of the NSAID, so it requires prolonged usage to have any advantage over, for example, acetaminophen. The bottom line is that even your use of over-the-counter pain medications should be carefully coordinated with any prescription medications in consultation with your doctor to balance the risks and benefits and to avoid overuse.

Following my back surgery, I was given a prescription for hydrocodone (synthetic codeine) with acetaminophen, to use on an ongoing basis for severe pain. Certainly, in a postsurgical situation, where pain is constant and severe, using such opioids can provide relief. For more episodic or occasional pain, I prefer trying other approaches to eliminate the pain rather than resorting to opioids, as the pain may change or disappear completely without introducing any narcotics at all. Nonetheless, there may be times when my pain is insistent enough that I rely on the hydrocodone as a last resort.

I have also occasionally taken prednisone (a steroid, cortisone derivative) for short periods of time when I have had persistent pain in my low back and legs of such severity that it is involving joints elsewhere in my body. The cortisone reduces pain and inflammation, and, with appropriate activity precautions and exercise, provides continued relief for a period of days to weeks. To me, this response is a

---

[35] Similar problems can occur with acetaminophen (Tylenol), which is also sold over-the-counter and compounded with other meds. Excess acetaminophen may cause liver damage.

testimony to the role the immune system plays in the expression and persistence of pain and inflammation.

Prednisone and cortisone derivatives can have some very serious side effects. I remember articles and pictures in *Life* magazine in 1949 where people severely disabled by rheumatoid arthritis were walking away from their walkers and wheelchairs because the newly available cortisone (then called *Compound E*) had taken away their pain.[36] It was a miracle. Further research, however, revealed that, in addition to more manageable side effects such as fluid retention, acne, and depression, prolonged and/or excessive cortisone use could have other more grave and irreversible side effects, including osteoporosis and suppression of the body's ability to fight infection.

Even after six decades of research and refinements, cortisone and its derivative medications (including prednisone) are still associated with many of these side effects. In cases where prednisone's risks are deemed to be outweighed by its benefits, its use must be judicious and closely supervised by a physician.

Pain needs to be addressed. It is telling us that something is wrong. The cause of our pain needs to be found and understood. Taking control of your pain issues will reduce the pain in the short-term as well as the long-term. If your pain is not controlled by measures outlined above or if your physician

---

[36] "Arthritis – Mayo Clinic Finds a Treatment for Man's Most Crippling Disease," *Life Magazine,* June 6, 1949, pages 104-113. "New Hormone for Arthritis: Drug from Hog Glands Supplements the Supply of Scarce Compound E," *Life Magazine,* September 19, 1949, pages 89-90.

does not feel comfortable treating your pain, you might consider consulting with a certified pain specialist.

Even with my training as a physician, as a patient, I am frequently embarrassed by the difficulty I have explaining the multiple locations, the varying degrees of severity, and different types of pain I am having. I can understand why it is very hard for a treating physician who does not understand polio and Post Polio to appreciate the variability of the pains as they relate to the diffuse nature of the neural/neuromuscular deficiencies. This is yet another reason why post-polio people should learn as much about polio and Post Polio as possible.

Chapter 11

Tiredness

For me, weakness came first, followed after a good while by pain. The third in the post-polio symptom trio was mental fatigue, or *tiredness*. Although in conversation the terms *fatigued* and *tired* are often used interchangeably, in discussing post-polio fatigue, it usually refers to the muscular fatigue – peripheral and central – associated with weakness, as discussed previously. For the purposes of this book, and for the sake of clarity, I will refer to mental fatigue as *tiredness*: a general state of weariness and exhaustion that affects the organism *as a whole*.

Tiredness and muscle fatigue work on different clocks. Muscles work twenty-four hours a day. The cardiac muscle is a perfect example; the muscle of our heart contracts seventy to eighty times a minute, more or less, for a lifetime. If properly paced, our skeletal muscles can go indefinitely as well. Even if we get out of pace and work our skeletal muscles hard enough to produce muscular fatigue, it will resolve in short order if the muscles are given a few minutes of rest to refuel and eliminate waste. Sometimes this muscular "resting" requires only a slowing of the pace, rather than stopping.

Tiredness, on the other hand, is cerebral and is far more

complex than muscular fatigue. It runs on the circadian clock used by the brain. The brain needs a seven- to eight-hour period of rest, which science now tells us is not really a "rest" period for the brain at all. In fact, it is quite the opposite. During this time, which usually comes in the form of a good night's sleep, the brain analyzes and integrates the newly acquired information of the day, making it more accessible for recall.

For the average adult on any given healthy day, seven to eight hours of sleep is typically adequate to alleviate tiredness. When additional tiredness is brought on by an acute illness, unusual stress, or simply the accumulated natural impacts of aging, more sleep may be necessary.

Two factors make it even more likely that those living with the late effects of polio will encounter significant tiredness. First, while polio has not been shown to cause depression in and of itself, the stresses related to living with post-polio weakness and pain may increase depression in those who are prone to it. Second, the increased mental energy required to accommodate for the disabilities left by the polio virus is a constant strain that can lead to tiredness.

Depression as a Cause of Tiredness

As I mentioned earlier, my first experience with post-polio tiredness came late in the game, after I retired. I had loved my work. My lifetime support groups had been my family, my office staff, and my patients (some of whom I had been seeing since I started practice in 1965). I lost daily contact with two of those three supports when I retired. For me, retirement was not the utopia found by others. I could not play golf or climb mountains, and the preparations to get out to fish were more tedious than the fun I could get from the sport. I went from a very comfortable and fulfilling professional life to a limited and dependent new lifestyle. So when I began to notice that I felt tired most of the time, I had to suspect that depression was playing a significant role.

Tiredness associated with depression is often a fairly persistent thing. It is not relieved by a brief nap as is muscular fatigue, nor is it responsive to a longer nap or overnight sleep, which may be adequate for the tiredness of sleep deprivation. With depression, one often wakes up as tired in the morning as when he went to bed at night. Tiredness that is prolonged and that is as severe upon awakening as it is at bedtime should be evaluated for depression, and if it is found to be depression, should be treated as such.

As I said, polio does not cause depression, but if one is predisposed to depression, life with Post Polio poses some additional challenges to fending it off. This is true both because the stresses and limitations of Post Polio can lead to despondency, and because some of the most physically active approaches to combating depression (e.g., a daily jog) are not readily available. When I retired, many of the ways that I had kept my life busy and satisfying – and had kept depression at bay – went away, and my post-polio situation contributed to (but did not cause) some depression and related tiredness.

The Strain of High Alert

The issue of tiredness came back at me with renewed

force after I broke my leg and has continued since then to some degree as I have dealt with increasing weakness and pain and collateral problems with my spine and mobility. This tiredness is representative of that to which post-polio persons (and others with significant disability) are prone. It is a mental thing. It is *a state of being weary*. One who is tired has used up a considerable part of his or her bodily or mental resources.

For those with Post Polio, tiredness results from the mental stresses related to the location and the severity of their paralytic polio. For example, my polio involves my legs, upper limbs, and, to a lesser degree, my trunk. Whenever I go anywhere new, I am preoccupied with whether I can get there, whether I will be able to get up and down the stairs, whether I will be able find a place to sit, and how I am going to be able to get back up again. Until I get settled and have those questions and a dozen or more others all answered, I am unable to relax and too distracted to make good conversation. Once I'm safely situated, comfortable, and have a getaway plan, I can relax and enjoy the company.

Many of the things that the non-afflicted do naturally, those of us with a polio disability may have to anticipate, calculate the risk of, and adjust for, long before implementation, and that takes energy. In high school, I had a part-time job sorting mail at the post office. I can remember that I would start adjusting the length of my steps twenty-five feet or so before I reached the stairway. That way, I'd hit the first step with my good right foot and grab the handrail at the same time to get me started safely and smoothly up those stairs.

So you see, our post-polio brains are constantly churning, working consciously and subconsciously to evaluate the alternatives available. What we did automatically before polio now requires forethought and considerably more energy. The mental vigilance that, by necessity, accompanies our disabilities is ever present – and it is tiring.

Chapter 12

Difficulty Breathing and Swallowing

As people age, they are more likely to experience difficulty with breathing and swallowing; this trend is a result of the natural attrition of aging. For those of us with Post Polio, whose attrition is superimposed on an already reduced neuromuscular mass, these difficulties are not only more common, but can pose a serious threat to our lives.

As will be discussed later in this chapter, while difficulty with breathing and swallowing is more frequently reported by those whose polio was diagnosed as bulbar polio, it is by no means limited to them. All polio survivors should be aware of the issues that can lead to difficulties in breathing and swallowing in the Post-Polio Stage.

Bulbar Involvement in the Acute Polio Infection

While I was being admitted to the hospital back on that fateful day in 1949, I remember overhearing an attendant ask the nurse, "Will he need an iron lung?" I had heard the term *iron lung* before, but I had never seen one and had no idea what they were supposed to do. As I was being wheeled down the hospital corridor, I witnessed two of the massive mechanical chambers and their captive occupants. I was relieved when the nurse replied, "It doesn't look likely he'll need one right now."

The nurses' initial concern regarding the iron lung arose because they understood from my parents that I'd had a sore throat and difficulty swallowing for a few days; with that history, they thought my polio might be of the bulbar type.

The *bulbar area* is at the top of the spinal cord, at the base of the brain. The area appears swollen, or *bulbous*, because of all of the nerves traversing it on their way to muscles in the chest wall, diaphragm, and upper extremities. From the bulbar area come the cranial nerves that supply muscles of the face and throat responsible for chewing and swallowing (the pharynx and larynx). Immediately below the bulbar area is the cervical spine whose nerves serve the neck and the diaphragm, and below that is the thoracic portion of the spinal cord whose nerves supply the rib cage.

As a result of the weakness or paralysis of laryngeal and pharyngeal muscles, bulbar polio patients were likely to have difficulty swallowing and impaired speech and be predisposed to aspiration of food and mucus into their lungs during the acute phase of their infection. In addition, because of the proximity of the bulbar region to the cervical (neck) and thoracic (chest) nerves, paralysis of the diaphragm and chest muscles often accompanied bulbar polio, affecting respiratory ability.

The iron lung had been invented twenty-one years before I got polio. Designed for the treatment of mechanical respiratory failure, it was a very basic machine. For those whose lives depended on it, confinement to the iron lung was constant. Caring for these patients involved reaching through holes in the sides of the chamber to perform the necessary tasks – bowel and bladder care, feeding, administering medications, turning the patient to prevent bed sores, and so on. The iron lung did a good job of pumping air in and out of the lungs, but neither the iron lung nor our understanding of respiratory physiology were sophisticated enough to handle the many problems that developed when the breathing and swallowing mechanisms were paralyzed for more than the briefest period of time.

You are beginning to see why in the 1940s and '50s the only diagnosis more frightening than one including the word *polio* was one including the two words *bulbar polio* – and rightfully so. Essentially, all polio deaths were associated with polio infection predominant in the bulbar area.

Fortunately, breathing or further swallowing problems did not play a significant role in the remainder of my infection. Because the weakness in my legs became my major polio symptom, it was decided that my polio was not the bulbar type, and I was given the diagnosis of spinal polio. It was not until well into the Post-Polio Stage that the many and varied problems associated with breathing and swallowing revealed themselves to me and to others whose paralytic polio had not been the bulbar type.

Post-Polio Difficulties in Breathing and Swallowing

We know that, by definition, in paralytic polio the polio virus penetrates the Blood-Brain Barrier and therefore has access to the entirety of the brain and spinal cord, including the bulbar area. So when they handed out diagnoses, the bulbar polio diagnosis was made only for those whose bulbar area had been so intensely attacked during the Acute Stage as to force prolonged paralysis of the throat and chest (often necessitating an iron lung). Otherwise, like so often in polio's game of give and take, those infected were considered "out of the woods," so to speak, and instead given a diagnosis of *spinal polio*.

It is only because of what we have learned through subsequent research that we now know that essentially everyone who had paralytic polio had some degree of bulbar polio – which explains why difficulties in breathing and swallowing are on the extended list of post-polio patient complaints, both for those who counted pharyngeal/laryngeal or respiratory involvement as a major feature of their acute infection and for those who did not.

Breathing

After the acute polio infection had cleared, I was left with little clinical evidence that the bulbar area had been infected. During my subsequent Recovery Stage, I played trumpet, sang in every kind of musical group in high school and college, and had no problem with breath control or stamina. My Stable Stage was much the same.

Now that my Post Polio is in full swing, however, I notice that bending over to tie my shoes or pick something up off the floor causes shortness of breath with very little provocation. My abdomen pushes up against my polio-weakened diaphragm, limiting its excursion and reducing my respiratory volume.

For those who suffered paralytic polio, the loss of nerve and muscle mass of the diaphragm and chest wall was much greater than anyone initially believed it to be. Fortunately, lung function is extremely efficient, so many suffered no outward signs of limitation throughout the Stable Stage. As we got deeper into Post Polio, some of us were surprised to find ourselves experiencing respiratory distress. We found that, when taxed by the stress of pneumonia, an asthma attack, a chest injury, prolonged surgery, or a hike in the mountains, difficulty breathing often ensued. Polio weakness of the legs and low back is not a direct threat to our lives, but polio weakness that involves our breathing muscles could be catastrophic.

The purpose of the lungs is to provide the body with needed oxygen and to remove carbon dioxide waste. The mechanics of respiration primarily involve movement of the diaphragm and rib cage. The diaphragm is made of skeletal muscle and gets its nerve supply from cervical nerves. The rib cage muscles are innervated by thoracic motor nerves of the spinal cord.

As the chest expands and the diaphragm flattens, the negative pressure created by these actions sucks air in. When inhalation has peaked, the chest and diaphragm muscles relax and an elastic recoil collapses the lung. In the process, the diameter of the windpipes (which had been expanded during inspiration) is now reduced. The reduction in diameter of the windpipes increases the speed and force of the air being expired, helping the cilia move mucus and foreign material up and out by blowing it toward the mouth for removal. This seemingly simple but phenomenal system is what maintains the cleanliness and health of our airways.

Ordinarily, breathing is one of the body's most efficient processes. Clearly, those who experienced respiratory distress during the acute polio infection had suffered serious injury to the nerve cells serving their breathing muscles. But even for those of us who did not have significant respiratory symptoms with the acute infection, if we are now experiencing respiratory distress with light to moderate activity in this post-polio phase of our lives, we can also assume there was a significant loss of neuromuscular mass for us as well.

Such reduced capability requires that special measures be taken to avoid undue demands on the respiratory system. First, concurrent or contributing conditions should be identified and eliminated or managed. For example, obesity, smoking, heart disease, and other issues need to be addressed proactively. Annual pneumococcal and flu vaccines are a priority; lung infections should be treated promptly. Snoring, sleep apnea, and other sleep issues should be checked out.

Some post-polio persons with breathing difficulties will benefit from ventilator assistance. Generally, supplemental oxygen is saved for use when other methods are not helpful.

It makes sense that we should work to preserve what

functional neuromuscular mass we have left in the chest wall and diaphragm. Do a few deep breathing exercises on a regular basis. Maintaining activity also serves to avert the mucus accumulation (and attendant windpipe obstruction, putrification, and inadequate oxygenation) that can come with disuse of the respiratory system.

Swallowing

Many of us were not aware of any *dysphagia*, or difficulty swallowing, until well into the Post-Polio Stage. Dysphagia is a result of nerve loss in the bulbar area. Although more commonly found in bulbar polio survivors, dysphagia, like the difficulty breathing discussed above, is a late symptom that may become obvious in post-polio patients whose acute polio infection was not initially considered bulbar. It is the result of accumulated weakness of the pharyngeal and/or laryngeal muscles – and this, we can see, is yet another example of the natural attrition of aging catching up to the end of our limited functional neuromuscular reserves in this area.

If you are noting problems from dysphagia – having trouble getting some foods to go down, choking or coughing while eating, or taking a long time to finish a meal – it is worthwhile to have a swallowing study done to identify which parts of the swallowing mechanism are giving you trouble. Sometimes non-polio-related issues may be causing or contributing to the difficulty.

Some approaches to managing dysphagia include dietary changes (limiting foods to those of a consistency that you can safely handle), special breathing or swallowing techniques (for example, adjusting the position of the head while eating), and adjustments to the timing of meals to avoid fatigue.

An Ounce of Prevention

As mentioned previously, everyone who has had paralytic polio should assume that they had some involvement of the swallowing mechanism and the muscles required for respiration. Even if you are not currently noticing problems with dysphagia or breathing, be alert to situations in which a lack of reserve capacity may put you at risk. For example,

- when other medical conditions arise that place extra demands on, or reduce the capacity of, your breathing or swallowing function;
- when your usual capabilities are diminished by fatigue, sickness, or alcohol or drug use; or
- when undergoing a surgical procedure that requires prolonged anesthesia.

In any of these situations, having a plan in place and sharing your polio history with your physician and caregivers can provide the proverbial ounce of prevention that is worth so much more than a later cure. If you have had polio, it would be a good idea, for example, to discuss it with your physician and anesthesiologist prior to any surgical procedure, as it may be necessary to assist your ventilation for a period of time after surgery until the anesthetic effect has worn off adequately. Such things as being able to force a cough to clear mucus-filled airways may require the availability of special equipment. All of the potential problems we have mentioned, and many others, are manageable if you and your team are prepared.

CHAPTER 13

FALLING

Falling is another hazard of aging that is a potentially greater risk for those of us in the post-polio population.

As a young kid, when I tripped, I would hop, skip, and jump a couple of times to regain my balance and then continue on my way. I might even take off on a brief run or do a few skips and whistle a few notes to show any onlookers that I wasn't hurting. After polio, during my Stable Stage, if I tripped, I might go stumbling forward for a few steps until I finally either gained control and walked away or fell to the ground. In those days, I still had enough strength and reflex to modify the fall so that, other than a hole in my trousers and an abrasion on my knee, I suffered little damage. But as Post Polio has led to more weakness and loss of reflexes, I am no longer able to quickly reposition my body to protect myself. The result has been a couple of nasty falls and some permanent disability.

Risk Factors and Falling

Falling is a progressively more frequent experience as we age, whether we have had polio or not. A 2006 article in *The Medical Clinics of North America*, reviewing the research on falls and the elderly, highlights this. In the older, non-polio population, falls are a major cause of death. In those over sixty-five, one out of three people fall each year. Falls are a major cause of sickness and death, and of the deaths that are due to falls in this country, about 75 percent occur in the small fraction of the population that is sixty-five or older.[37]

Oddly, the risk of death or long-term disability following a fall does not necessarily result directly from the fall itself but may be more attributable to the prolonged rest time required to heal. Such inactivity can contribute to the development of pneumonia, kidney failure, heart failure, blood clots, or sepsis. So although the death certificate may list one of these as the cause of death, the precipitating event may have been a fall.

As we age, falls are likely to be multifactorial, meaning they were caused by a combination of both intrinsic risk factors (i.e., related to the individual) and extrinsic risk factors (i.e., related to the environment). In reviewing sixteen independent studies of risk factors in falls, the *Medical Clinics* article identified nine intrinsic risk factors that at least doubled the odds of falling. These included (starting with the greatest increase in risk):

- Lower extremity weakness
- History of falls
- Gait deficit

---

[37] Laurence Z. Rubenstein, MD, MPH, and Karen R. Josephson, MPH, "Falls and Their Prevention in Elderly People: What Does the Evidence Show?" *The Medical Clinics of North America*, 90 (2006): 807–824.

- Balance deficit
- Use of assistive device
- Visual deficit
- Arthritis
- Impaired activities of daily living
- Depression

You will recognize many of these risk factors from earlier discussions in this book. Although they are clearly characteristics that become more common as people age, many of them are inherent symptoms of Post Polio. At the top of the list is lower extremity weakness, which studies found increased the odds of falling on average by more than four times. The next three factors on the list – history of falls, gait deficit, and balance deficit – approximately tripled the odds. All of these factors are likely to be present in any post-polio person, especially those in whom polio affected the lower extremities.

Post-Polio Limitations in Breaking a Fall

Even if, with years of polio experience, polio survivors have learned to be more cautious to mitigate some of this increased risk, when they do fall, the consequences are likely to be more severe than a similar fall in a non-polio peer.

A while back, after a visit, my granddaughter came running at me unexpectedly with a good-bye hug and kiss. She barely reached me, but the surprise was enough to start me tipping backward. And down I went, with my head, neck, and back landing flat as a board. I landed so hard that I actually bounced a little bit, but I couldn't see that I was injured. I looked to my right through the grass and saw a sprinkler head projecting six inches out of the flower bed. I was only inches from being impaled on that sprinkler!

My granddaughter was so frightened that she ran back into the house. For me, it happened too quickly to get scared, but I remember it as the weirdest of experiences. I did not have a cane or walker, and there was nothing else for me to grab to break or prevent my fall. I didn't collapse or crumble. My knees didn't even buckle. I just tipped over, as if I were a pole. I've thought of that fall, the sprinkler head, and the dreadful potential a thousand times since then.

What impressed me the most was how completely unresponsive my muscles had been to my crisis. The weakness in my legs tethered me so I could not change the position of my feet. The weakness in my abdomen, neck, and the core muscles of my back and sacrum prevented me from curling up to protect myself, especially my head and neck. Similarly, when I fall forward, although my knees may buckle, I cannot activate my leg, back, and neck muscles to modify my position or abort the fall. The powerful reflex impulses, which are the first to recognize danger and come to our rescue, cannot activate muscles that are too weak to respond. Fortunately, I still have enough strength and reflex in my arms to extend them to break a forward fall.

Preventing Falls

Thanks to safety research and advocacy, we have the benefit of legislation providing curb cuts, elevators, uniform step heights, lighting standards, handrails, and other fall-preventing features in our communities, to name only a few. Never neglect to take advantage of them. Use handrails, grab bars, or a walking stick when available. Pay constant attention to where you are going and what type of surface you are walking on. Precautions like these will go a long way in helping to avoid injury and disability.

When you first looked at the table of contents of this book, you may have asked yourself, "Why a whole chapter on falling?" Now you know: falls are a real threat to our lives, a threat that is with us at every turn and with every step we take. You must never, knowingly, put yourself in harm's way. Observe, plan, and then make your move.

Chapter 14

Exercise

As I bring this book to completion, I am quite limited physically. Now in my late seventies, I have been wearing braces on my legs for the most recent third of my life and have had three spinal surgeries in the last four years. An athletic twenty-something would probably get quite a kick out of the idea of me writing a chapter on "exercise." But his idea of exercise and mine are not necessarily the same.

For me, exercise is not limited to marathons, tennis matches, spin classes, and the like. I refer to exercise in the broad sense: "(1) regular or repeated use of a faculty or bodily organ; (2) bodily exertion for the sake of developing and maintaining physical fitness."[38] Any movement or activity that helps us to improve or maintain our health and range of function should be considered exercise for us as survivors of polio.

And, given that definition, the truth is that exercise is one of the few tools that we have available to modify or control the progression of our Post Polio, decrease pain and fatigue,

---

[38] *Merriam-Webster's Medical Dictionary*, s.v. "exercise," accessed February 25, 2011, via Dictionary.com, http://dictionary.reference.com/browse/exercise.

maintain productivity, and improve our sense of well-being. Therefore, it is important that we understand it and even more important that we embrace it.

Disuse, Overuse, and Finding the Right Balance in Your Exercise Program

In a 2003 "Statement about Exercise for Survivors of Polio," members of the post-polio medical community articulated the benefits of therapeutic exercise for polio survivors, while emphasizing the importance of moderation and individualization to avoid overuse that can cause damage to the joints and muscles.[39] A complete exercise program should be developed with the collaboration of a physician and, ideally, be under the initial direction of a professional with post-polio expertise.

If you currently have an active exercise program, hopefully you are already aware of and adhering to the existing guidelines for exercise and Post Polio, including using low to moderate intensity, slow progression of exercise, pacing with adequate rest intervals, and a rotation of exercise types. For additional suggestions and guidance, you may wish to look at the following resources:

---

[39] Medical Advisory Committee of Post-Polio Health International, Martin B. Wice, Chair, "A Statement about Exercise for Survivors of Polio," *Post-Polio Health* 19, no. 2 (Spring 2003); also available at http://post-polio.org/edu/pphnews/BrochExercise.pdf. The statement was also endorsed by twenty-nine other members of the post-polio medical community.

- ***Non-Fatiguing General Conditioning Exercise Program (The 20% Rule)*** – A moderate approach to exercise by Stanley K. Yarnell, MD. (*Available at* www.post-polio.org.)[40]
- ***Reap the Rewards of Post-Polio Exercise*** – A fact sheet and resource summary from the National Center on Physical Activity and Disability. (*Available at* www.ncpad.org.)[41]
- ***Sit and Be Fit "Post-Polio Exercises" webpage*** – Exercise guidelines and references to suggested "Sit and Be Fit" videotape workouts for polio survivors. (*Available at* www.sitandbefit.org.)[42]

But if you do not have an exercise program, and – because you've always had the same idea of exercise as the athletic twenty-something – you thought you could never exercise again, this chapter may help you to see how you can begin to make your own version of exercise become part of your life, regardless of your physical limitations.

---

[40] Stanley K. Yarnell, MD, "Non-fatiguing General Conditioning Exercise Program (The 20% Rule)" Post-Polio Health Vol. 14, No. 2 (Spring 1998), http://www. post-polio.org/edu/pphnews/pph14-2d.html.

[41] Sunny Roller, MA, and Frederick M. Maynard, MD, "To Reap the Rewards of Post-Polio Exercise," *The National Center on Physical Activity and Disability*, updated 2007, http://www.ncpad.org/disability/fact_sheet.php?sheet=136.

[42] "Post-Polio Exercises," *Sit and Be Fit with Mary Ann Wilson*, accessed February 26, 2011, http://www.sitandbefit.org/postpolio.

What an Exercise Program Should Do

An exercise program should aim to do several things: (1) increase strength and endurance, (2) improve fine motor coordination, (3) enhance flexibility, and (4) discourage the development of osteoporosis.

Increase Strength and Endurance

Perhaps it goes without saying that our exercise program should strengthen the body with the goal of maintaining and improving on the function and abilities we still have. We know that for us, as polio survivors, becoming world-class athletes is not likely, so it is foolish to design our exercise routines or measure our strength in those terms. Exercise should be approached with the understanding that we have a reduced functional neuromuscular mass and that we need every bit of strength possible to retain function for the activities of daily living. We should exercise to attain and maintain levels that will sustain that.

Improve Fine Motor Coordination

In addition to maintaining and increasing strength and endurance, an exercise program should also be designed to improve muscle coordination and enhance fine motor skills. To do this, slow, controlled movements need to be incorporated into the exercise routine. Neurologically, such movements are very sophisticated, reflecting input from every area of the body and mind, interpreted by millions of individual muscle fibers.

Enhance Flexibility

Our program should also include stretching exercises to keep muscles limber and viable. Muscles and tendons tighten up after periods of disuse or misuse. This tightening may adversely affect the short- and long-term mechanics of muscles and joints. If tightening is extreme, over time the muscle's contractile tissue may be damaged and permanently replaced by fibrous scar tissue. This is referred to as a *contracture*. Contractures can be very disabling because they restrict movement, and attempting to move a muscle in contracture may be painful. Pain can discourage us from exercising and stretching, which in turn can lead to weakness and further tightening.

Discourage Osteoporosis

Osteoporosis is a thinning of bone due to loss of its calcium. On a microscopic level, bone is constantly building and remodeling, shifting the balance of *osteoblasts* (bone cells that use calcium to build bone) to *osteoclasts* (bone cells that break the bone down). Because the number of osteoblast cells tends to decrease as we age, osteoporosis is prevalent in the elderly, especially in those who are not physically active and whose diet is lacking in calcium. The bone thinning of osteoporosis increases the ease of fracture, which, especially for those of us with Post Polio, can be detrimentally life changing.

Weight bearing, as in walking or running or any other activity that requires you to support weight, stresses the bone. This load stress on the bone stimulates the production of osteoblasts, which in turn pull calcium into the bone to strengthen it. This explains why osteoporosis is an issue for the astronauts, whose in-space weightlessness deprives them of normal weight-bearing opportunities, and for those who are bedridden or confined to a wheelchair for a length of time. It is one of the reasons why your doctor wants you up and on your feet as soon as you are able after surgery or an illness.

Osteoporosis is a major concern for many restricted by Post Polio, especially those affected in the lower extremities. To the extent possible, an exercise program should include weight-bearing exercises designed to discourage osteoporosis.[43]

Basic Concepts of My Exercise Program

Satisfying all of these goals is a tall order, and it is important that each of us work with our healthcare professionals to find a program that is right for us. Exercise had never been a part of my daily routine in my younger years, and by the time my Post Polio caught up with me, my physical abilities were so restricted as to make most "normal" forms of exercise unavailable to me. I had to get creative.

The approach I will lay out is only an outline, which you may elaborate upon and tailor to your strengths, weaknesses, and capabilities. I would emphasize that this program is mine, and it works for me. It is not intended to replace an effective program you already have. But for those of you to whom the

---

[43] Additionally, with your physician's consultation, you may wish to explore not only daily calcium supplements but also the new drugs designed to put calcium back into bone.

idea of exercise seems foreign and out of reach, my program illustrates how someone with significant polio-related physical involvement incorporated exercise into his daily routine – and greatly improved his quality of life.

Two seemingly unrelated examples of exercise served as the inspiration for my program: swimming and Kegel exercises – go figure. Let me explain.

Swimming: The First Inspiration

When movements have been modified by paralysis or weakness, there may be many viable muscles that are not being used. For instance, the weakness in my lower extremities from polio renders me unable to squat, pick up paper from the floor, run up the stairs, and more. Because of the restrictions of movement resulting from my paralysis, I have dozens of squatting, lifting, and bending muscles that are rarely used, and without work, they weaken and atrophy. If I can strengthen these unused or little-used muscles, the increased strength will help stabilize my joints and their movements, and with this will come an increased sense of physical and mental well-being.

Swimming is a perfect exercise for strengthening unused or little-used muscles. The buoyancy that occurs when we are submerged in water results in a reduction of our effective weight by about 90 percent. This works to our advantage: An otherwise immovable extremity in a polio person, when submerged and buoyed, may be movable by the weakened post-polio muscles, giving those muscles a chance to be used and strengthened.[44]

When I was still practicing medicine full-time, the problem with swimming, for me, was that it took me about thirty minutes to get my clothes and leg braces off and then another thirty minutes afterward to get them back on. I was spending over an hour just getting in and out of the pool (not to mention the time to get to and from a pool), and right or wrong, I didn't feel I could afford that much time. Yet I had learned that the weightlessness effect I experienced in the water was essential and needed to be included in my exercise program.

I found that I could accomplish much of the non-weight-bearing benefits of swimming by exercising in bed. While lying down, the buoyancy effect of the mattress allowed me to do lots of exercise movements for my legs and back that I could not do while standing or sitting – exercises I could otherwise only do in the water. I refer to these as my *swimming-in-bed* exercises. As you'll see, swimming in bed is especially easy to adapt to provide slow movements for coordination and stretching for improved flexibility and range of motion.

It was when I looked to find ways to work more on strength building that I came upon my second inspiration.

---

[44] If you have access to a pool, try performing a series of movements in five feet of water and then try them again in the shallow end. Those of you with marked leg weakness will notice that, when you are submerged to the neck and shoulders, you may be able to do all kinds of kicks, flexions and extensions, and toe stands. But when you are in the shallow water, you may have a return of pain and weakness that necessitates your clinging to the edge of the pool to support yourself and relieve the pain.

Kegel Exercises: The Second Inspiration

While practicing medicine, I occasionally prescribed Kegel exercises for patients with urinary incontinence and other problems related to a weak pelvic floor. As you may be aware, a Kegel exercise involves squeezing the pelvic floor muscles to strengthen those voluntary muscles surrounding the urethra that help control urine flow from the bladder. To properly perform Kegel exercises, you must first identify the right muscles and then learn how to voluntarily contract and relax them. When refining your Kegel technique, you will be instructed to focus specifically on your pelvic floor muscles and to take care not to contract other nearby muscles such as those in your abdomen, thighs, or buttocks.[45]

The effectiveness of the Kegel comes from concentrating on isolating one muscle group at a time and finding a way to contract and release that muscle group to build its strength. It does not require equipment, videos, mobility, or even that anyone else be aware that the exercise is being performed. So while the Kegel is specifically designed to address the muscles of the pelvic floor, it occurred to me that the same approach could be applied to exercising other muscles, including the abdomen, thighs, and buttocks – those that are expressly excluded when you are trying to do a proper Kegel!

You might understand this best if you do it with me right now. So, start with a proper Kegel: squeeze down on the pelvic floor muscles enough so you could stop urine flow.

---

[45] You'll also be told that, once you've got the technique down, you should do at least three sets of ten or fifteen ten-second contractions a day.

Now, go beyond the Kegel, squeezing a bit harder so that the abdominal muscles are tightening. Now a third time, squeeze harder still and note that the inner muscles of your thighs are tightening as well as the abdominal and pelvic floor muscles. The fourth time, squeeze even harder so that the buttocks muscles are contracting too and are actually digging into the seat of your chair.

When you do these Kegel and "beyond-Kegel" exercises, you voluntarily contract the pelvic floor muscles, the abdominal wall muscles, the adductor muscles in your thighs, and the gluteus maximus in your buttocks. All of these muscles are skeletal. You can voluntarily contract every skeletal muscle in your body this same way.[46] With such isometric contractions, when the muscle is contracted, there is tension, but no shortening or lengthening of the muscle.

Giving the Concepts a Try

Again, for those of you who already have an active physical fitness program in place, the concepts that I've laid out are likely to seem quite rudimentary and unnecessary – and for you, at this time, they probably are. If you are already involved in a well-rounded exercise routine that is tailored to

---

[46] As noted previously, there are three types of muscle: (1) cardiac or heart muscle; (2) smooth muscle that lines the gut, bladder, and stomach; and (3) skeletal muscle. We have no direct control over cardiac or smooth muscle, but we do have almost complete control over skeletal muscle. Therefore, exercise activities need to be directed toward strengthening and improving the coordination and efficiency of our skeletal muscle.

your lifestyle and takes into account your polio involvement and post-polio considerations, you are not in need of advice about how to get started with exercise.

But for those of you who have felt so physically restricted or confined that you believe exercise is outside the realm of possibility for you, perhaps the concepts of swimming in bed and the beyond-Kegel isometrics have helped you to realize that all of us can find ways to develop an exercise program.

Also, recognize that simply increasing your activity can be the start of your exercise program. At this time, there is an image I would like you to place in your mind. Think of a baby in a crib. As you imagine that baby, note that hardly a second goes by that there is not some degree of movement – kicking, churning, crying, grinning, or other physical activity – going on in that baby's life. That is how a baby develops his strength and coordination, whether in the womb or in the crib. By contracting many muscles at once, as in a fitful crying episode, or a few at a time, as with a grin, a baby develops, strengthens, and matures his neuromuscular system. Every time you watch a baby, use him as an instructor; notice the frequency and the variable intensity of his movements. You will be learning from an expert, and it won't cost you a cent!

What I would like to have you do now is to try playing with the concepts a little bit. Whether you are lying in bed or relaxed in a chair, practice contracting every muscle you can find, starting at the top of your head and marching down to the tips of your toes. First, try using short contractions, and pay attention to the fading retraction (relaxation) after each contraction. Then try it with more intense contractions. Try varying your position. If you are in bed, do some exercises while on your back, side, and abdomen. While on your abdomen, with your feet hanging over the edge of the bed, pull your toes forward against the end of the mattress repeatedly to exercise the dorsiflexor muscles. Weakness in these muscles is associated with foot drop.

Now try grouping the muscles by region: the lower extremities, upper chest, shoulders and arms, abdomen, and pelvis. Then try some generalized contractions. (For me, the most impressive accomplishment of my swimming-in-bed exercises is that I am able to flex and extend my hips and knees, which I can do while lying on my side. I can't even budge them while sitting or standing.)

At this point, you might try adding music. If you decide to exercise to music, you will be listening to it over and over again, so using music that will inspire you is important.[47] I use an iPod with earplugs. This way, I don't disturb my wife or anyone else. Music provides a rhythm to follow. More importantly, repeatedly exercising with music will help develop a conditioned response, so, like Pavlov's dogs, when you hear your exercise music or similar trigger, you will automatically start your isometric exercises, or at least be reminded to do them.[48] After a couple of months, you will find that the sound of music invites you to exercise, whether you're in the car, in a chair – any place and any time.

---

[47] My daughter reintroduced me to Anne Murray, a Canadian singer with a clear, beautiful voice, and for me, the perfect rhythm.

[48] No, you should not start salivating. If that happens, you are doing it wrong, and I suggest you start over.

The exercise program should include some movements to work on the coordination and fine motor activity of the neuromuscular system. These are the slow, controlled movements and stretching that I referred to at the beginning of this chapter, and they come more easily to me when I am enjoying some music. I also think of the elderly Chinese doing their Tai Chi exercises; their movements are very controlled and sophisticated. This type of exercise is especially important for the upper extremities.

Try it now. For example, slowly and smoothly outstretch your arms with palms down. Now, cross your arms, with the upper arms crossing midway between the elbows and shoulders. With this, you are gently stretching the shoulder muscles. Continue this position, but with the palms turned up. Note that simply changing from palms down to palms up affects which muscles are contracting and which are relaxing. Now, with both hands, pretend you are reaching for a cloud. Pull it to your chest. Break it in two and put it back again. Pay attention to which muscles you are using. Be creative. While maintaining control, vary the speed and intensity.

A Cautionary Note

If you watch late-night TV or spend time on the Internet, you have likely been bombarded with ads for fertility products, cheap loans, imitation Rolex watches – and exercise devices. If you have ever considered investing in one of these exercise products, or in any one-size-fits-all exercise device, be aware it was probably not developed with a post-polio user in mind.

We are different from our non-polio peers – very different. For example, one major difference is that polio involvement is rarely symmetrical. One of those exercise devices may have a function that would work for one side of your body, but not for the other. Just be cautious. And because they were really not designed for the likes of us, using them as designed might not be an option for you.

In Conclusion

Those of us with Post Polio are at high risk of decreased function due to muscle disuse. When one is hurting, disabled, tired, or weak, it is so easy to invite disuse in as a friend. But disuse is not a friend. The swimming-in-bed exercises are especially helpful in the treatment and prevention of disuse atrophy because they can be used by anyone with almost any degree of disability.

While disuse is our enemy, it is important to remember that overuse can also have a detrimental effect on polio survivors. The proper balance between exercise, rest, and the activities of daily living is an equation that will look different for each of us and ultimately should be calculated in consultation with your health professionals.

I hope you can now see how my exercise concepts can be a starting point for building your own program to exercise unused muscles and introduce an exercise routine into your daily life. In my case, I used them to begin working toward the goals of increasing strength and endurance, improving coordination, and enhancing flexibility that I discussed at the beginning of this chapter. For the fourth goal, discouraging osteoporosis, I rely primarily on daily walking, as in my situation that constitutes weight-bearing exercise.

Since beginning my swimming-in-bed and beyond-Kegel exercises, I have continued to expand my repertoire as my strength and capabilities have allowed, with occasional periods of retreat when surgery or other setbacks have required it. I have added light hand weights and Therabands. In preparation for my most recent surgery, I worked with a trainer and have continued to work with him and a physical therapist after the surgery. I feel strongly – and my doctors agree – that this exercise contributed greatly to my recovery.

CHAPTER 15

WEIGHT CONTROL

For anyone who is overweight, there are a myriad of benefits that result from reducing your weight to a healthy and optimal level. For those with Post Polio, the benefits of eliminating excess weight are especially significant.

Excess weight takes a toll on our weight-bearing joints.[49] The lower extremities and back were designed for weight bearing, with more muscle, bigger bones, and a distinct, supportive, musculoskeletal structure. Unless we are lying or sitting down, the back and lower extremities must bear the entirety of our body weight while either maintaining its position or moving it wherever the brain demands.

In contrast, the joint structure and bone design of our upper extremities are intended for throwing, pushing, pulling,

---

[49] If you would like to study the effects of excess weight on gait, structure, and performance, go to the airport. You can learn a lot as you watch people of varying sizes walk those long walkways. Note how little extra weight it takes before someone starts to waddle; it places a different angle of stress on the knees, hips, and feet. Note, too, that the bigger the belly, the greater the sway in the back. These positional changes stress the muscles and injure the weight-bearing joints. It is the same for everyone, but lugging around unnecessary body baggage is especially damaging to our weakened post-polio bodies.

and performing fine, detailed movements. Those of us who were left with weakness in our legs find that we must use our arms for lifting the weight of our bodies up and out of chairs or bed. These maneuvers – which are performed dozens of times per day – put an abnormal strain on the hands, wrists, elbows, neck, and shoulders and can lead to deterioration in the upper limb joints and pressure-type neuropathic injuries, as seen in carpal tunnel syndrome.

The results of such deterioration and injuries – damage to the joint surfaces, abnormal stresses on the supportive tendon and ligament structures, the resultant stress on the muscles, and pressure on various nerves – trigger pain and discomfort. Unfortunately, by the time this pain is first felt, the joint has probably already been damaged. As you can see, the likelihood and magnitude of such damage proportionately increases with the amount of excess weight that someone carries.

Calories Count

Over the years, I have had many, many patients ask me about the merits of various popular diet programs. If they were hoping to hear me sounding like a celebrity spokesman for one or another of them, they were sorely disappointed. As far as I'm concerned, there is no magic in the Atkins Diet. The people living in South Beach are not better cooks than you are, and there are a lot of fat people in California and Florida who have had grapefruit growing in their backyards for years. The simple truth is that you will not lose weight on a diet unless the number of calories you absorb on it is less than the number of calories you burn. The variable is really *you*. Will you stick to it, and how will you feel while you are doing so? You can develop a diet plan that will work for you if you understand a few basics. You won't have to read a book, but you will have to read labels.[50]

The calories we ingest come in the form of carbohydrates, proteins, and fats. There are four calories in each gram of carbohydrate, four calories in each gram of protein, and nine calories in each gram of fat. When it comes to weight loss, it is basic math: a calorie absorbed is a calorie gained. However, not all calories are created equal, and the differences are what make a particular eating program easier or harder to follow.

Carbohydrates are absorbed very rapidly, especially the simple carbohydrates in foods made with processed and refined sugar, which have very little nutritional value other than their caloric energy. Within one hour after their ingestion, the blood sugar rises. Depending on the type of food and amount of carbohydrate ingested, the blood sugar may rise enough to precipitate the release of an excess amount of insulin, which may in turn bring the blood sugar down quickly and often too far. If the blood sugar is dropped too low (hypoglycemia), it can produce a sensation of hunger, often associated with a feeling of anxiety caused by the body's release of adrenalin. The adrenalin releases glucose from the glycogen stores in the liver in an attempt to get blood sugar levels back to normal. With the "empty" simple carbohydrates in processed and refined sugars, we get calories, but

---

[50] The calorie counts that the government now requires on all food labels makes counting calories a snap.

they don't stick around long enough to satisfy our hunger. And by stimulating the release of excess insulin, they may actually increase our hunger. This is not really something you want in a weight-reduction diet. The simple carbohydrates in fruits, vegetables, and milk products (which provide important vitamins and minerals) and the complex fibrous carbohydrates such as those in legumes, grains, and starchy vegetables (which are slower to be absorbed and generally contain more nutritional value than their simple counterparts) are the better choices when choosing carbs.

Fats are absorbed slowly. They may take two to six hours to be fully absorbed from the digestive system. In addition to the slowness of the chemical process, fats slow the motility of the stomach and intestines. Both of these factors help to give us a feeling of fullness, or *satiety*. Fats also give food a pleasant texture. On the flip side, fats have over twice as many calories per gram as proteins or carbohydrates, so it is important to monitor your fat intake when trying to cut calories.

Proteins fall somewhere between fats and carbohydrates as far as absorption speed is concerned, usually taking about two to four hours to be absorbed into the system. Not only are proteins responsible for tissue construction and maintenance, they are also very satiating, which makes them the key player in a weight maintenance program. Both fats and carbohydrates are energy sources for the body, but proteins are vital metabolic building blocks – so adding eggs, poultry, meats, and other protein-rich foods to your diet is essential.

It is no secret that much of the rise in obesity in America may be tied to the increased use of processed, refined sugars and other non-fibrous carbohydrates over the decades. Cutting back on these low-nutrient simple carbohydrates is where we should start when reducing calories. Fats should be limited to 20%–35% of our daily caloric intake, and proteins should be pushed to 10%–35%. Fats and proteins will give you the greatest feeling of appetite satisfaction, and that in turn will give you the best chance of sticking to your diet.

Usually, when I start a weight-reduction program, the first thing I notice is that my shoes are too big. We almost always lose more weight in the first few days of the diet than we do in the second week. That's because the first things that happen when we significantly reduce caloric intake are a loss of water and an adjustment in the amount of material stored in the bowel, which make it seem as though we are losing a lot of weight.[51] We are, but we're not losing fat, just fluid and stool. It is a good idea to wait until the body has made these adjustments before we start evaluating the effectiveness of a diet. The fluid in the tissues and the material in the bowel will return to normal as soon as we settle into the new, lower-calorie regimen. Then you will see how much true body weight you have actually lost.

Dr. Leff's Egg and Toast Diet

About thirty-five years ago, I was frustrated by patients who would "swear to God" that they were not eating more than a thousand calories per day and still were not losing weight. I knew they were not counting calories correctly

---

[51] In fact, many proprietary diets include a diuretic element to amplify their apparent weight loss.

because there is no way you cannot lose weight on a thousand calories per day. To test and challenge them, I came up with the *Egg and Toast Diet,* as follows:

- Egg on toast, three servings a day (four times a day if the patient is large and active), each consisting of:
    - One fried egg (about 85 calories)
    - One level teaspoon of butter or margarine to be used on the toast or to fry the egg (about 35 calories)
    - One slice of toast (about 85 calories)
- Unlimited water and no-calorie beverages
- Unlimited cucumbers, lettuce, celery, zucchini, raw carrots, and fresh tomatoes
- (Optional) Low-calorie salad dressing of less than 15 calories per tablespoon, if desired, but not exceeding four tablespoons per day

Three servings of egg on toast total about 615 calories per day. Add the vegetables and dressing, estimated at 160 calories, and you are at 775 calories, still well below the 1000-calorie mark. My dieters followed this exclusively for three weeks, at which time we would evaluate their weight loss and decide whether to continue with the diet a bit longer. Usually, they continued with a modification of the diet based on what we'd learned; then, once the desired weight was achieved, they changed to a maintenance plan based on desired weight, activity, blood sugar, cholesterol levels, etc.

Most people found the Egg and Toast Diet to be filling,

quick and easy to prepare, and relatively well-balanced nutritionally, with a fixed number of calories. Certainly, one could cheat by using larger bread and eggs and higher-calorie dressings, but anyone who would do that probably wouldn't be sincere enough to follow the program for the length of time it required.

The diet was not meant for the long term, but rather to show my patients that they *would* lose weight on 700–1000 calories per day. Many elected to continue on this diet until they reached their goal. My sister-in-law stayed on the diet for six months until she lost the fifty pounds she'd wanted to shed. My daughter used it for three weeks to lose the ten pounds that were bothering her. Many Egg-and-Toast-Diet alums still use it periodically, going back to it if their weight begins to increase. I have Egg and Toast as my breakfast meal.

I initiated this diet in the 1970s, and it worked beautifully. But shortly thereafter, the news media became concerned about the connection between dietary cholesterol and incidents of heart attack and stroke and pointed a finger at eggs as the cholesterol culprit. Though I disagreed with the anti-egg hype, I backed off on prescribing it to my patients. However, for years, people called back asking me to remind them of the details of the Egg and Toast Diet.

I should say that four eggs per day, when incorporated into a strict low-calorie diet, will not increase the serum cholesterol. The cholesterol levels we checked on patients on the Egg and Toast Diet showed a marked decrease in serum cholesterol, never an elevation. Actually, the purpose of a weight-reduction diet is to burn fat from your fat stores; therefore, in reality, any time *you* are on a strict, low-calorie diet, you have put your *body* on a high-fat diet.

How Much Are You Burning?

Once you have followed a low-calorie diet for a period of time, there is a simple calculation you can use to estimate the number of calories you are burning each day.

- First, determine the number of calories ingested during the period of the diet. Take the number of calories ingested in a twenty-four-hour period and multiply that by the number of days of the diet (or if you are not using the same number of calories each day, simply keep track of and total the number of calories used over the period).
- Use the number of pounds lost to determine the additional number of calories burned by the body during that time. To do this, multiply the number of pounds lost by 3,500 calories.
- Add the two numbers together and divide the total by the number of days of the diet, and that should give you the number of calories used per day at your current level of activity.

As an example, let's use the Egg and Toast Diet outlined above. Let us say that on this diet I was eating a fixed 775 calories a day, and in the second and third weeks of my diet

I lost a total of five pounds.[52] By multiplying 775 calories times fourteen days, we know that I ingested 10,850 calories during those two weeks. In addition, my body also burned five pounds of fat to sustain itself for a total of 17,500 calories (five pounds times 3,500 calories). By adding 17,500 to 10,850, we know that I burned 28,350 calories. If we divide those 28,350 calories by fourteen days, we calculate that I was burning 2,025 calories a day.

Once you've done the calculations, you can use this information to customize your weight control program. To increase the rate of weight loss, you can increase your activity. Alternatively, if you were finding that the amount of caloric intake was not sustainable for you, you could increase it to 1,000 or 1,200 calories per day, accepting the fact that your weight loss would be more gradual. And if you have eliminated all your excess weight and are now at a healthy weight for you, you would then know how much you could eat at your current level of activity to maintain the status quo.

Tips for Success

Because calorie restriction is not a lot of fun for the majority of us who have problems keeping the excess weight at bay, it is important to do what you can to make it as painless as possible. Over the years, my patients have related a variety of tricks they have used to help them "stay the course," and I'll share some of those here with you.

---

[52] In the first week, I lost four pounds, but we'll disregard that week because we know it includes water and bowel weight loss that are temporary.

- Limiting your food intake does not have to mean making mealtime miserable. Some of my patients found that enhancing the dining experience – whether with music, table linens, or the company you keep – made them miss the food less. It's possible to create an experience that is high on aesthetics and low on calories.
- Avoid nibbling and other uncounted food consumption. Put excess food away after setting the proper portions on the table to reduce the temptation to finish off the casserole or have a second helping. Clear the table immediately, put away leftovers, and wash the dishes to squelch some of the urge to nibble as you clean up.
- Plan ahead what you are going to do as soon as you are finished eating so that you have something to focus on and, hopefully, look forward to once your meal is complete.
- Instead of a glass of wine or dish of ice cream, celebrate life's events with non-caloric choices such as going to a movie or taking a walk in the park.
- Check your weight often and keep a running record of it, and use a journal to track your food intake. People who do this seem to fare much better than others, not only at keeping to the rules of their eating plan but sticking with their plan for the duration.
- Memorize the calorie count of as many foods in

your diet as you can. Having this information in your head makes it easier to estimate and anticipate caloric intake and to make the inevitable trade-offs that will be required when life throws you a curve ball on the menu.

So what have we learned? (1) If you are carrying excess weight, your post-polio body will benefit greatly from safely eliminating it as soon as you can. (2) The most important thing to remember in organizing your weight-loss plan is that calories do count. If you plan your meals for nutritional balance, estimate the calories needed to accommodate the activities of the day, and reduce your calorie intake and increase your activity to a level that you burn more calories than you absorb, you will lose weight.[53] You have to motivate and dedicate yourself, but it will be worth it.

---

[53] Include a good daily vitamin with minerals and micronutrients and a separate supplement of 1–2 grams of absorbable calcium as well. Don't megadose on vitamins; it never is a benefit and may cause serious problems.

Chapter 16

Self-Advocacy and Post-Polio Support

I hope that reading this book has increased your knowledge of what happened to your body during your long-ago polio infection and what is happening to it now. That knowledge should give you the confidence to serve as your own best advocate when it comes to health and quality-of-life issues.

Your post-polio body is not like every other aging body that goes through your doctor's office, into your retirement center swimming pool, or out to bridge club with the gang. You should not expect that what works for your non-polio friends will necessarily work for you or that they will understand that it won't. You are the expert on your own body and should not hesitate to pursue answers and solutions when you suspect that post-polio issues are impacting your health or well-being.

Take the Lead:
Help Educate and Focus Your Team

When you look for answers and solutions, you may find that your healthcare professionals and/or family and other caregivers are not aware of the unique issues of Post Polio: you must take the lead in bringing them up to speed. Encourage them to read books (including this one!) and articles, to refer to websites, and to contact experts as appropriate to ensure that your post-polio considerations are not overlooked in your healthcare management and decisions.

Even after you have placed your polio history and post-polio concerns firmly on your doctors' radar screens, you should continue to check in with them about any specific issues or concerns as they arise. Don't be bashful or hesitate to double-check, as Post Polio is not a common enough condition to presume that every medical professional is fully versed in all its ramifications. For example, if you are anticipating surgery, you will want to confirm that the surgical team is aware that your polio history may influence your respiration and recovery from anesthesia.

Proceed with Caution: Snake Oil and Anecdotes

I don't think I have ever met with a post-polio support group where someone didn't ask about the healing effect of some herb, oil, or special diet they had heard about or other anecdote. It appears that the snake oil salesmen are still around.

Now that you better understand the physical aspects of polio and Post Polio, you should have an advantage over most people in seeing through some of the sure-cure sales pitches. I, too, would like to find something that would help me have less pain and fatigue, more strength, and get my thirty-two inch waist back. But I so often see that the product they're pitching just can't live up to the hype, that I can't encourage anyone to even try it.

I am, however, very much a believer in nature's remedies.[54] Very few of our effective drug therapies were designed from scratch, without using some natural therapeutic compound as a starting point. Most of the designing that is done today is done to improve on the therapeutic chemical compounds already provided by nature so that they may be better absorbed, have fewer or more tolerable side effects, reach a broader spectrum, and so on. So it's not nature's remedies that concern me; it's those treatments and so-called "cures" that feed on our desires but are not based on valid research or science that I worry about.

For example, I'm always a bit skeptical when I hear about a product that will not only cure all my ills but, more importantly, "doesn't contain any chemicals." (Everything is chemicals. Nature is chemicals!) And I am similarly cautious about anecdotes of successful treatments such as "Jeannie told me her Uncle John had been soaking his sore knees in Mexican beer for the past three weeks and now his pain has

---

[54] For example, digitalis came from digitalis leaf (commonly called foxglove), and many of our other current medications originally came from plants or animals or bacteria or fungi. More than forty years ago, I visited the Eli Lilly Pharmaceutical Company in Indianapolis. They showed me a very large warehouse where they had stored and carefully catalogued thousands of plants, seeds, animal parts, and the like, to study their possible therapeutic effects. The pharmaceutical industry still has people searching for plants, bacteria, fungi, and animals that might contain or produce a chemical compound that could be used therapeutically to treat diseases. I believe that nature is the ultimate biochemical and genetic experimenter.

gone away." Here we have secondhand, unsupported, anecdotal information about a cure for sore knees, and most of us would greet this story with justified skepticism.

We need to know what caused John's knee pain, how long he had it, and how the beer solution was administered. We should know how warm the beer was and whether it was applied with gentle massage. Was there any simultaneous change in John's other medications or activities? During the course of the beer therapy, did he happen to throw out a pair of shoes that was putting abnormal stress on his feet and knees? Was he still pain-free at the end of the two months? Was the beer the active ingredient or would warm water soaks and massage produce the same result (without wasting good Mexican beer)?

The importance of verifying the validity of a promoted cure or therapy cannot be stressed enough. You must consider the source, do your homework, and confer with your doctors to ensure that it will not interfere with your current regimen or pose other risks.[55]

---

[55] I know the wife of an elderly diabetic patient who took him to a community about one hundred miles from home to consult with her herbalist. The herbalist immediately took the patient off his insulin and other support medications and placed him on a concoction he had prepared. The patient went into a diabetic coma and congestive heart failure and died before he could get back home. Had they checked out the proposed concoction and coordinated with this gentleman's physicians before going to the herbalist, it is possible that his life could have been saved.

Find Strength in Numbers: Post-Polio Support Groups

So far, I have focused on how to advocate for yourself when those around you are not familiar with the unique issues and challenges you face with Post Polio. It can feel somewhat daunting and maybe even a little lonely. Participating in a post-polio support group is a perfect antidote – placing you in a community where you are part of the majority, instead of the minority. Here, you are able to relax and draw support from others who are experiencing the same concerns and many similar manifestations as you.

A post-polio support group provides, among other things, the opportunity to share resources, hear from experts, and work together to develop a helpful lexicon for communicating with your non-polio team members. Many of us with polio developed an incredible self-sufficiency over the years and find the dependency that Post Polio necessitates to be difficult to handle; sharing these unique difficulties with our post-polio peers can help us both to develop strategies for accepting the help we need and to recognize the value we can provide in supporting others.

As independent, self-sufficient individuals who have coped with the impacts of polio over the years, many of us have come up with unique strategies, systems, and workarounds to make our lives easier. A support group provides an opportunity to share with and learn from each other and to appreciate the ingenuity of our peers.

Shortly before retiring, I joined a post-polio support group. After attending it and visiting several others, I became aware of how little professional advice or support was available to those of us with Post Polio. The local polio support groups have done a marvelous job of educating and supporting group members as well as educating the political and medical communities. To find a post-polio support group in your area, you can do an Internet search for "post-polio support" or go to Post-Polio Health International's website (post-polio.org) for a list.

Optimize Your Post-Polio Life: A Review

At the beginning of this book, I told you that I hoped my twin experiences as a polio survivor and a physician would be of benefit to you as a reader. I hope that this book has helped to take some of the mystery out of the medical aspects of polio and Post Polio, and to give you a context for the advice and accommodations you will come across in the future.

Perhaps it is ironic that, despite all the medical foundation I've tried to provide, the most significant things that each of us can do to improve our lives with Post Polio are within our personal (non-medical) control. I realize that, for the rest of my life, my degree of happiness, productivity, and physical stability will be in large part the result of my own commitment to:

- Support my weakened structure with necessary bracing, recognizing that excessive bracing could lead to disuse atrophy.
- Avoid "moments of stupidity" or otherwise putting myself in harm's way.

- Pace myself with regular nighttime sleep and intervals of rest between periods of activity.
- Exercise appropriately and on a regular basis to maintain and improve function.
- Maintain my weight at an ideal level to put the least stress possible on my muscle and bone structure.
- Maintain an active partnership with my medical team, family, and caregivers to coordinate my health and quality-of-life issues.
- Connect with available post-polio support networks to empower and sustain me in my post-polio challenges.

These things are not expensive and do not involve special medications. They are simple and realistic – and require effort, desire, and a will to optimize our lives now and for as long as we live.

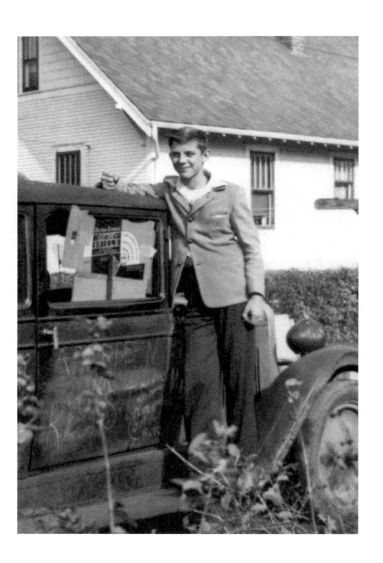

ABOUT THE AUTHOR

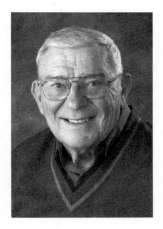

Wenzel A. Leff was born and raised in Mobridge, South Dakota, the third of six children. After graduating from medical school at Washington University in St. Louis, Missouri, he began a long and active practice in Internal Medicine. Dr. Leff and his wife Julanne have called Pullman, Washington, home for over forty-five years.

Since retirement, Dr. Leff has pursued his interests in travel and healing with medical mission trips to Ecuador and researching and writing about Post Polio. He divides his time between Pullman and Seattle, Washington, enjoying friends, family, and especially his ten grandchildren. This is his first book.

INDEX

Accommodation, 77, 88
Acetylcholine, 39, 113
Acute pain, *see* Pain
Acute polio infection, *see* Polio, Infection
Acute Stage, 33-35, 38-40, 61-70, 77-78 (*see also* Polio, Infection)
Adenosine triphosphate (ATP), 125-130
Allen, D. G., 129
Anecdotes, 202-203
Anesthesia, 30, 140, 164, 202
Antibiotics, 9, 21, 75
Antibodies, 52, 56, 65, 67-68, 103-105
Antigen, 56, 66-67
Apoptosis, 80-82, 109
Arthritis, 87, 144-146, 148-149, 169
ATP, *see* Adenosine triphosphate
ATPase enzymes, 126
Attrition, *see* Natural attrition of aging
Axon, *see* Nerve

Back surgery, 27-30, 134, 142-143, 148, 173, 187

Balance
   Coordination, 24, 92, 167, 169
   Electrochemical, 78-80, 83, 107-108
Beijerinck, Martinus, 47
Bellinger, Andrew M., 133
Beyond-Kegel exercises, *see* Exercise
Blood-Brain Barrier (BBB), 53-55, 61, 98, 102-104, 160
Braces (leg), 19-20, 23-24, 35, 88, 123, 180, 206
Brain, 38, 51, 53-54, 58, 82, 108, 124, 130-132, 134, 138-139, 151-152, 158, 160
Breathing, 8, 36, 71, 118, 120, 157-159, 160-163, 164
Broken leg, 22-24, 87-88
Bulbar area, 7-8, 158-159, 160, 163
Bulbar polio, *see* Polio

Calcium (Ca2+), 78-79, 107, 129-130, 133, 177-178, 199
Calories, 190-199
   Burning, 191, 196-197, 199
Capsid, 49, 51
Carbohydrates, 191-193

Cashman, Neil R., 37
CD155, 51 (*see also* Polio virus receptor)
Central muscular fatigue, *see* Muscular fatigue
Central nervous system (CNS), *see* Nervous system
Cleanup Phase (of Recovery Stage), 76, 77-82, 85, 106-107
Clinical Phase (of Acute Stage), 63-64
Complement system, 66
Compound E, 149
Contractures, 9, 177
Cytokines, 69, 145-146

Depression, 30-31, 134-135, 145, 149, 152-153, 169
Difficulty breathing, 8, 36, 118, 120, 157, 160-163, 164 (*see also* Breathing)
Dimmock, Nigel, 47
Disuse, *see* Muscles
Dr. Leff's Egg and Toast Diet, *see* Egg and Toast Diet
Drugs, *see* Medications
Dura, Miroslav, 133
Dysesthesia, 140
Dysphagia, 163-164 (*see also* Swallowing)

Easton, Andrew, 47
Egg and Toast Diet, 193-196
Electrochemical levels, 77-80 (*see also* Balance, Electrochemical)

Exercise, 9, 24, 28, 34, 55, 77, 86, 95, 143, 146, 173-187, 207
   Beyond-Kegel exercises, 182-183
   Kegel exercises, 179, 181-182
   Program, 34, 95, 146, 174-185, 186-187
   Swimming in bed, 180, 183-185, 186-187

Falling, 23, 167-171
Fat, 126, 128, 191-193, 195-197
Fatigue (generalized), 36, 53, 63, 91, 120, 145, 151, 164, 173-174 (*see also* Tiredness)
Fine motor coordination, 176, 185
First Research Symposium on the Late Effects of Poliomyelitis, 21-22, 119 (*see also* Warm Springs Conference)
Flexibility, 176, 177, 180, 186
Footpads, 39-41, 111, 113, 132
Fracture
   Blood-brain barrier, 54, 98, 102
   Bone, 22-25, 177
Functional neuromuscular mass, *see* Neuromuscular mass

Gait, 92, 168-169, 189

Glia, 83, 104, 106-108, 110-112

Halstead, Lauro S., 22
Hog glands supplements, 149
Hogle, James, 49
Hubbard tub, 9, 73, 75
Hubbell, Susan L., 37
Hyperextension, 19, 20 (*see also* Recurvatum)
Hypertrophy, 76, 85-86 (*see also* Muscle, Building)

Immune response, 64-68, 70, 77, 78, 80-81
Immune system, 52-53, 56, 61, 64-68, 70, 77, 78, 80-81, 105, 145-146, 149
   Adaptive *vs.* innate, 64-65
Immunity, 46-47, 56-57, 100, 102-105, 112, 145-146
Immunization, *see* Vaccination
Immunological memory, 65
Impulse(s), *see* Nerve
Incubation period, 34, 62-63, 67-68
Infantile paralysis, 5 (*see also* Polio)
Inflammation, 54, 65, 68-70, 79, 98, 102, 108, 139, 140, 145-146, 148-149
Inflammatory response, 65, 68-70, 78, 80-81, 145-146
Iwanowski, Dmitri, 47

Josephson, Karen R., 168

Kegel exercises, *see* Exercise
Kenny, Sister Elizabeth, 8

Lännergren, J., 129
Late effects of polio, 21-22, 37, 48, 118-121, 152 (*see also* Post Polio and Post-polio syndrome)
Leppard, Keith, 47
Life Magazine, 149
Lymphocytes, 56, 67-68, 80, 104-105

Memory, 56, 67-68
Macrophages, 66-67, 77, 80-81, 103-106
March of Dimes, 48, 120
Maynard, Frederick M., 175
Medical Clinics of North America, 167-168
Medications, 30, 53, 58, 141, 147-149, 164, 178, 203
Memory lymphocyte, *see* Lymphocytes
Mendelsohn, Cathy, 50
Moments of stupidity, 24-25, 206
Monocytes, 66
Muscle
   Building, 75, 85-86, 180-182
   Disuse, 9, 24, 28, 86, 142-143, 174, 177, 186, 206
   Fiber types, 84, 87, 95, 124-127, 128-129, 182
   Fuel, 126, 127-130

Muscle (*continued*)
   Orphaned muscle fibers, 34, 40, 42, 43, 76, 81, 82-84, 110, 112-113
   Overuse, 174, 186
   Skeletal, 124-125, 129, 130, 142, 151, 161, 182
Muscular fatigue, 117-118, 123-135, 151-153 (*see also* Weakness)
   Central, 124, 132, 134, 151
   Peripheral, 124, 134, 151
Myelin, 38-39, 41, 83, 84, 109-110

National Center on Physical Activity and Disability, 175
National Institute of Neurological Disorders and Stroke, 120
National Institutes of Health, 120
Natural attrition of aging, 44, 91, 95-96, 118, 144-145, 157, 163
Necrosis, 80-81, 102, 108
Nerve, 7, 10, 34, 35, 37-44, 55, 64, 76, 78-84, 93, 96, 106-113, 119, 135, 140-141, 143, 145, 158, 161-163
   Axon sprouting, 34, 41-43, 76, 82-84, 96, 109-111 (*see also* Reinnervation)
   Impulse, 38-39, 82, 111, 124, 130-132
   Regeneration, *see* Reinnervation
Nerve cell adhesion molecule (N-CAM), 83, 113
Nervous system, 35, 53-54, 56, 61, 82, 97-108, 131, 145
Neuromuscular mass, 36, 43-44, 93-96, 124, 134-135, 144, 157, 162-163, 176
Neuromuscular reserves, 36, 91, 92-95, 142, 163, 164
Neuropathic pain, *see* Pain
Node of Ranvier, 41
Nonsteroidal anti-inflammatory drugs (NSAIDs), 141, 147-148

Oligodendrocytes, 107-108, 112
Optimization Phase (of Recovery Stage), 76, 85-89
Orphaned muscle fibers, *see* Muscle
Osteoporosis, 23-24, 149, 176, 177-178, 187
Overuse, *see* Muscles

Pacing, 126, 151, 174, 207
Pain, 22, 35-36, 43, 64, 68, 79, 87-88, 91, 117-118, 120, 135, 137-150, 151-152, 154, 173, 177, 180, 190
   Acute, 127, 138-139
   Neuropathic, 140-141, 143
Paresthesias, 140

INDEX

Peripheral Disintegration Model of PPS, 37
Peripheral muscular fatigue, *see* Muscular fatigue
Phagocytes, 66, 104-106, 111
Plasma cells, 67, 80, 104-105
Point of maximum recovery, 15-16, 18, 35, 72, 75, 77, 85, 89, 91-92, 94, 138
Polio, 5-6, 18, 31, 33-34, 38-40, 44, 45-59, 61-70, 81-82, 86, 92-93, 119, 157-160, 163-164
   Bulbar, 7-8, 157-159, 160, 163
   Infection, 6, 33-35, 38-40, 42, 61-70, 93, 96, 157-159, 160, 162-163 (*see also* Acute Stage)
   Research, 48-49, 50-51, 57-59, 118, 119, 160
   Spinal, 8, 159, 160
   Survivors, 1, 22, 31, 35, 42, 44, 48, 71, 85, 86, 88, 91, 92-94, 117-119, 123, 157, 163, 169, 173-176, 186
   Virus, 7-8, 9-10, 37-38, 45-59, 61-68, 70, 77, 81-82, 97-112, 117, 160
Polio virus receptor (PVR), 50, 51, 55, 58, 63, 112
Poliovirus, *see* Polio, Virus
Post-Polio Health International, 38, 174, 175, 206
Post-Polio Stage (Post Polio), 22, 31, 33-34, 35-36, 38, 42-44, 59, 91, 96, 117-121, 123, 124, 132, 135, 137, 142, 143, 150, 153-154, 157, 159, 161-162, 163, 167, 169, 173-174, 177-178, 186, 189, 202, 205-206
   Support, 11, 201-207
   Symptoms, 31, 35-36, 91, 117-120, 135, 151, 159, 163, 169
Post-polio syndrome, 22, 31, 35, 37, 42-43, 59, 119-121, 123, 142
Post-Polio Task Force, 37
Pre-Clinical Phase (of Acute Stage), 62-63 (*see also* Incubation period)
Prednisone, 148-149
Protein (in foods), 191, 192-193

Racaniello, Vincent, 50
Recovery Stage, 15, 33-36, 41-42, 71-89, 93-94, 160
Recurvatum, 20, 24, 87 (*see also* Hyperextension)
Reiken, Steven, 133
Reinnervation, 9, 34, 36, 37, 41-44, 76, 82-84, 85, 94, 96
Reinnervation Phase (of Recovery Stage), 76, 82-84
Remodeling, 76-77, 85, 86-88, 177

Research, *see* Polio
Reserves, *see* Neuromuscular reserves
Ribonucleic acid (RNA), 49-52
Roller, Sunny, 175
Rubenstein, Laurence Z., 168

Sabin vaccine, *see* Vaccination
Salk vaccine, *see* Vaccination
Schwann cells, 83-84, 110-111
Self-advocacy, 119, 201-207
Sister Kenny Treatment(s), 8-10
Sit and Be Fit, 175
Skeletal muscle, *see* Muscle
Spinal polio, *see* Polio
Stable Stage, 33, 35, 41-42, 91-96, 160-161, 167
Strength, 9, 12-13, 85-86, 95-96, 124-125, 143, 176, 178-182
Support groups (post-polio), 11, 205-206
Swallowing, 7-8, 63-64, 118, 120, 157-160, 163-165
Swimming in bed, *see* Exercise

Tiredness, 43, 70, 117-118, 134-135, 145, 151-155

Vaccination, 48, 55, 56-57, 65, 68, 103, 112, 117, 162
  Sabin vaccine, 55-57
  Salk vaccine, 56-57

Warm Springs Conference, 21-22, 119 (*see also* First Research Symposium on the Late Effects of Poliomyelitis)
Weakness, 8-9, 16, 19, 22, 26, 30, 35-36, 43-44, 64, 73, 87, 91, 93, 117-120, 123-135, 142-144, 145, 146, 151-152, 154, 158, 159, 161, 163, 167-170, 177, 179, 180, 184, 190, 206
Weight (weight control), 19, 88, 146, 189-199, 207
West Nile virus, 42
Westerblad, H., 129
Wice, Martin B., 174
Wiechers, David O., 22, 37
Wilson, Mary Ann, 175
Wimmer, Eckard, 59

Yarnell, Stanley K., 175